How to
Be a Thin
Person

How to Be a Thin Person

Raysa Rose Bonow

With an Introduction by
Dr. Gerard Musante

Random House New York

Library of Congress Cataloging in Publication Data
Bonow, Raysa Rose.
How to be a thin person.
1. Reducing diets. I. Title.
RM222.2.B618   613.2'5   77-3579
ISBN 0-394-40616-8

Manufactured in the United States of America
2 4 6 8 9 7 5 3
First Edition

For
Mom and Dad
love and "bite"

Introduction

I am sure that many readers of *How to Be a Thin Person* are aware that Durham, North Carolina, is a well-known weight-reduction center in the United States. As a result of her participation in our program in Durham, the author has written this excellent book, which allows everyone, no matter where they live, to share and understand the experience of the structured-behavioral weight-control program.

How did this approach develop and why can *How to Be a Thin Person* be helpful to you? To answer this, let me list some facts which research on obesity and clinical observation have demonstrated.

(1) There is no medical treatment for obesity. There is no drug that will have long-term effectiveness in weight control.

(2) There is no diet or magic combination of foods that will let you lose weight quickly or easily. People do not stay on diets very long without interruption, and the guilt attached to so-called "cheating" triggers feelings of depression and worthlessness, which in turn only trigger increased eating.

(3) Treatment of obesity by drugs and fad diets fails because the patient lapses back into his former habits and eating behavior.

If you have failed in the past, both you and your physician, perhaps even your family and friends, probably considered this proof of your lack of self-control, or your lack of character, etc. Actually, "will power" and character have very little to do with weight control, as you will discover when you read this book.

This book is based on the premise that in such cases of failure perhaps it was the *treatment* itself and not you that was to blame.

How to Be a Thin Person is based upon principles of behavior psychology, and views obesity as a learned addictive behavior disorder. Eating disorders are intractable because they are learned behaviors, habits practiced and strengthened over a period of years. Eating provides immediate positive reinforcement, temporarily relieves anxiety and for many provides a major source of life's gratification. Therefore, effective weight control requires that you change your eating habits and your life style, not just go on a diet for a few weeks and then return to the old behaviors that caused you trouble to begin with. Also, you must learn to alter the fundamental importance of food in your life so you will not have to always diet to stay thin. *How to Be a Thin Person* illustrates the re-education process necessary to enable you to learn appropriate eating habits and food-related behavior.

Why is the concept of environmental control so important? Studies on obesity have shown that people's eating habits are influenced by various things. For example, time, visibility of food, the social situation, stress and boredom. Hunger plays only a minimal part in eating problems. It is the other influences in the environment which cause the most difficulty. Discovering the particular problem, place, person, situation and time which cause you the most problems is the important first step toward making necessary changes in behavior.

I am particularly glad the author has so extensively covered the topic of eating out. She skillfully applied what she had learned here about structuring her food environment to many new and different situations. Each of you, if you keep the diary as suggested, can measure your behavior and pinpoint the time, food, person or situation which triggers your overeating. You can then begin to plan a strategy *ahead of time* which will help you handle situations better. This is what structuring is all about—using the environment for your benefit so that, as the author states, you are no longer "the victim of special occasions."

One of the most important principles of behavioral psychology is that of positive reinforcement. Praise, not punishment. No one likes failure. That's why *How to Be a Thin Person* encourages you to shape your behavior, to take small steps at a time and to make small changes. Each little success gives the courage to continue until the ultimate goal is reached. It would be unrealistic to expect you to give up your old habits all at once. It would be unrealistic to expect that you will never deviate from your structured menu. In Chapter VII, The Cycle, the author outlines the small steps to alter the act of eating. Each is a specific and achievable target behavior. The important principle of learning to remember is that occasional failure does not impede successful behavior change. The important thing is that the desired behavior occur more frequently than not from day to day; occasional breaking the diet or "unstructured eating" is not catastrophic.

I cannot tell you that *How to Be a Thin Person* will work perfectly for everyone, or that reading a book will allow you to treat yourself. I can assure you that all of the systems in this book are based on principles of psychology, and that the overall philosophy is the result of several years of observation and treatment for over 1,500 patients.

Sometimes you will not be able to carry these systems out. When that happens, they still serve a purpose. That is, they tell you that some situation needs further work for which you may need to see a professional. As you learn to structure your food environment, and change your life style, it is reassuring to know that the author did it, and that you too can learn How to Be a Thin Person.

Dr. Gerard Musante
Clinical Director of Structure House
Center for Weight Control and Lifestyle Change
707 Morehead Avenue
Durham, North Carolina 27707

Acknowledgment

At a very critical time of my life, I happened onto some good fortune and was able to spend some time at Duke University Medical Center under the sensitive counseling of Dr. Gerard Musante, who is now continuing his extraordinary concepts at Structure House in Durham, North Carolina.

What I found out there was that "I had a right"! They told me so, and it took me quite some time to believe them. They started me thinking, and because of the thinking, I found the person I had left behind a long time ago.

On the path to rediscovering myself, I realized that one cannot always live in a diet-structured environment, such as existed at Duke; that one has to live in the real world.

Their initial input led me to know that:

I had a right to my feelings.

I had a right to express my feelings.

I had a right to expect certain things from certain people.

I had a right to live the life I wanted.

Starting to realize all these very simple concepts made me desire to put them down on paper. This book is the result of my thinking. I hope it helps you find what you're looking for.

Thanks again to Dr. Musante ... and to Dr. Sigrid Nelius at Duke ... for showing me that I could have hope.

To a very special couple who volunteered to live the concepts of this book before it was even a gleam in my eye. Having lost the weight they needed to lose, they continue to enjoy the regimen today, and I am ever grateful to them ... my loving and lovely Mom and Dad, Esther and Samuel Bonow.

To my friend Joan Shiel, who was the first to believe that this was a book that should be written.

To the friends who read early pieces of the manuscript and encouraged me to continue on this new path ... Francine Achbar, Pearl Bromberg, Lisl Cade, Allyn Claman, Leonore Commora, Vicky Cooper, Don Cornelius, Martha Cotioux, Saya Feldman, Charna Garber, Patsy Geller, Gail Granik, Edith Pinero Green, Kenny Jacobson, Joyce Kahn, Glorianne Katz, Esther Margolis, Raysa Oker, Dorothy Papush, Howard Papush, Caroline Wean and my sister, Mary Lou Finesilver ... thank you!

To my editor, Charlotte Mayerson, whose superb sense of "the word," honed and shaped and exposed the heart of my manuscript.

Special thoughts to my dear friends Richard Taylor and

Clay Cole for their confidence in me and their constant support.

And to all the people everywhere who carry more than their extra weight with them: I've written this book for you.

You Don't Have to Be Fat Any More . . . or Ever Again!

I have done them all—Weight Watchers, Dr. Atkins, Dr. Stillman, pills, pink pills, blue, green, the cholesterol diet, the "eat all the bacon you can swallow" diet, the shots-every-day diet. And I was successful on all of them. On each, I lost about twenty-five pounds (when I needed to lose fifty), and each time I started to look good or "better" I relaxed and put back all the weight . . . and a little more.

No one, including my doctor, ever told me how to take it off and keep it off. I have been there—up and down—my entire adult life and, finally, I have made it! The most important thing I can do now is share my experience with you and help you as others have helped me and as I have learned to help myself!

I know what it's like to have the tray not come all the way down in the airplane because my stomach is there. I know what it's like to be terrified of the summer and the beach and showing everyone my "grotesqueness." I know the humiliation of barely fitting into the seat in the theater, of having the seat buckle hardly buckle, of squeezing my heart out to get the zipper to the top, of seeing a wardrobe of every size in my closet, of deciding not to look in the mirror any more—not below the neck anyhow —certainly not in any store window I passed.

Even while I was writing this book there were small detours, but now, with what I know, they are only detours, and in a moment I'm speeding right down the highway again. I'm in control of me now! You can be in control of you! You have a right to a life free from such torments.

Diet is not the only answer, although this book provides a wonderful one. The answer is that food cannot be separate from the rest of our lives. We can't diet in isolation! What we're talking about here is how to have a new life from this moment on, to have food in it, but not to be all of it. What I will try to do is to provide you with a survival course through all the possible dangers . . . from hunger pangs in the morning to a business luncheon in a fancy restaurant, to attending a baseball game, to going to a wedding or having Thanksgiving at your home.

I know how helpful, and how detrimental too, family and friends can be. We'll talk about that. I want to share it all with you. I know you'll understand every word.

I understand you . . . you are me and I am you.

Few doctors can ever understand our heads, no matter how hard they may try. Put the doctors aside for a moment and let's sit down together and share our lives. Our humiliations, our sadnesses . . . that's yesterday. Yesterday is over. Our successes, our hopes, that's TODAY, and with these new todays, our tomorrows will be what we always wanted them to be.

You are a good person. You have just probably forgotten how to be kind to yourself. And until you begin to be kind to you, you can't get anyone else to be kind to you!

This time, this diet, is the last one you're ever going to be on. Because this is no diet, this is a new life.

We'll talk about how to cope with restaurants, parties, even the circus. We'll learn how to deal with husbands, wives, children, parents, sisters, brothers, friends, business associates.

We'll talk about structuring your day. TIME ON YOUR HANDS IS FOOD IN YOUR MOUTH!

We need help and we need support. I have devised support systems, because when you're a person who has decided to be thin, you need lots of supports: a good scale, a diary, a calorie book, a good walk, some delicious time for a rest.

You will find out that, no matter what, you're never a failure. The only failures in this world are the ones who have given up. As long as you keep trying, you are a success or on your way to success.

There is only today and the thought of tomorrow. There are no recriminations for yesterday. There will be no more accidental meals or accidental fatteners left hanging around our shelves.

We will know what we will eat, how we will eat it, where we will eat it and when. We will know with whom we will share our meals and our life. We will find out that we are entitled to insist upon a new planned healthy life.

And for the first time in our lives, we will know what real hope is. We will discover that we are in control and are not victims of anything . . . any place . . . any person!

xvii

Contents

How to
Be a Thin
Person

I Never Thought
I Could Do It!

This book is not about how I lost weight. There is no point to that, and it would be no favor to you to go over my day-by-day experience. The problem is not: "What is the diet?" "Exactly what do you eat?" These are the first impatient questions from most people. Probably most of you know how to stay on a 700- or 1,000-calorie diet, and if you need help you will find such a diet on page 111.

What we all need to know is how to change the ways we used to lose weight, so that this is the *last* time any of us will have to do it. How can we change the way we approach food so that life can be more than the constant negative attention we have to pay to our bodies? How can we deal with food *and* with life in a way that is worthy of the really wonderful people we are?

This book is for you, whether you're suffering with the constant five or ten pounds you can't seem to deal with, or whether your goal is a much larger one. The problem is the same . . . the pain and suffering are the same . . . the solution is the same.

Each of you can live a fantastic, wonderful life with love, friends and food and be a thin person. I thought I would never be able to control food, but I have learned to change every conceivable way in which I approach food . . . from thinking about it, to buying it, to preparing it, to eating it . . . to throwing it away. It's a simple solution, but until we apply these ideas over and over again, they have no use. It's Pavlovian, and we ourselves are the dog as well as the bell.

If we keep repeating our behavior, one day it will become as automatic and natural to us as it is to a thin person. We will no longer be at the mercy of food. We will be in control. We will be walking a tightrope.

There is a doctor in Philadelphia who has been repatterning children who have been brain damaged—moving their arms and legs twenty-four hours a day—making the brain understand new thoughts that perhaps it never knew. That is what must be done. We must start all over again.

More likely than not, you have probably *never* known how to deal with food in your life. There is no point in asking why. Why is it that any of us take the wrong path? Perhaps . . . perhaps it may have something to do with the way you were fed as an infant. Perhaps your mother fed you too fast . . . too slow. Perhaps she fed you when you wanted . . . perhaps when she wanted. Any combination of these factors—no point. We're not talking about the past. We're talking about today and the years ahead for you, how to have lunch today, how to make dinner for you and your family tonight, how to live the years to come with food in its proper place, as something we deal with three times a day, enjoy, share with friends and

4

family. But that's all. The period between lunch and dinner should not be overrun by thoughts of what you won't eat that night. What *will* I eat tonight, when no one is around?

Once you have control of this program, the period between meals will be calm and productive because you won't have to think about food at all. Just imagine! Your meal is planned. It's written down. The preparation is done. The food is in the refrigerator. You know what you will eat and you can be calm about it because you thought it out yesterday. You know you won't eat until dinner because you are someone who doesn't eat between meals.

WHAT A RELIEF!!!! Try that on. Say it with me. "I am a person who doesn't eat between meals." "I am a person who doesn't eat between meals." This is one of the commandments for life. The rest are in the following pages. You won't understand fully what each one means, but we're going to go into them as we move on our way through the program. We'll take enough time so that you are able to use them as your own. Copy them out for yourself. Read them again—over and over. Put one in your wallet, one on your refrigerator door. One in the center of your dining-room table. One in the bathroom, if that's where you do your thinking.

The Commandments

(1) I am a person who eats three meals a day.

(2) I am a person who does not eat between meals.

(3) I am a person who eats at the same place in my house every day.

(4) I am a person who plans my meals at least one day in advance.

(5) I am a person who writes down my meals and also my unstructured eating.

(6) I am a person who plans my day.

(7) I am a person who is kind to me.

(8) I am a person who is not a victim.

(9) I am a person who weighs myself every day.

(10) I am a person who takes a good brisk walk every day.

(11) I am a person who must crawl before I can walk . . . who must walk before I can run . . . and must run before I can fly!

Chapter 1

Take My Hand!
It's Time to Begin
a New Life!

Now, are you ready to begin that diet? Though we all want to wait for the perfect time to begin a diet, there is no perfect time. It will never happen. There will always be a wedding around the corner, or Father's Day, or your birthday, or the Christmas office party, or the jitters over a relationship, or the once-a-year picnic at Robert's farm. The special days and nervous moments continue round and round like a merry-go-you-know-what, never ending, never stopping. Now. This is the perfect time to start living a healthy, happy, calm, productive, thin life. Look at your watch. Mark the time and date down right there. Write it in this book. Use this book as a tool to help you get what you've always wanted in your life and maybe you didn't know it . . . and that's control. Control over your own life. You are no longer going to be a victim. You are going to be kind to yourself. You have an absolute right to your claim to get the most out of this life. What is it that you want? A good job, good grades, a husband, a wife? All those things are easy. All those things will come when you're in control.

Think of the energy we waste in constantly worrying about being thin. Think of the anxiety we often feel before eating or after eating what we shouldn't. Think of how we feel when we deprive ourselves of what everyone else is having.

That anxiety is a kind of reverse energy. It's sapping your strength. It's making you tired. It's making you feel you can't achieve anything. It's an energy that should be rushing from you toward other things, other ideas—expanding, relieving, calming and pleasing you. Instead, it is making your body feel as though it weighs a million pounds. You don't want to feel like that, but we all know what you do when you feel that way. You eat!

Why? Because food is really calming. Stop: reread that sentence. *Food is really calming.* The body calms down when the food gets in, but only for a moment—cloaking briefly the constant anxiety you're feeling because you are out of control. You hurt and you suffer because of your fatness—regardless of how many pounds that represents and because the things you really want do not seem attainable. So you have learned the great delusion. "If I eat, I will feel better. It will all go away." It is that terrible chain of events we are going to work together to stop.

Let me tell you a story.

One day I was in my car, driving to a restaurant to have dinner. A terror hit me so suddenly I almost lost control of the car. I began to perspire because—I found myself thinking that I had already eaten! But how could that be? I had just left my house and was on my way to dinner. How could I have eaten . . . unless the act had been so traumatic that I had blocked it out? My brain went rushing over the day's events, and I tried to re-create that moment when I felt the panic and tried to remember what I had been thinking or feeling just before it. All I remembered was that I was calm. CALM! I was calm. It took me a while to unravel it . . . but what I found out was so incredibly simple and so majestic in meaning for me that I am almost afraid to talk about it.

I believed that if I was anxious and I ate, I would feel better. But then I would hate myself for eating, feel anxious again and eat again to calm myself down. Dieting made me anxious, and my brain had begun to equate "dieting" with "feeling anxious."

Now, let's go back to me in the car. I'm on a weight reduction program. I should feel anxious, but I don't. I'm calm! So, for a moment, my brain read CALM, and that meant I must have just eaten! WRONG! What I was feeling was the way most people feel when they are in control or are getting in control of their life and their problems. If we could think of unplanned food, food that we hadn't planned to eat, as a fix, like a shot to a drug addict, or a drink to an alcoholic, we certainly wouldn't view it as good positive action. Why do addicts behave the way they do? For the same reason that you eat: because they have relieved their anxiety, momentarily. They then feel the same guilt and dislike for themselves and take another drink, another cigarette, a fix.

We could live out our days relieving our anxieties with the very thing that we're anxious about—but the body doesn't like it that way. It gets tired, worn out with the abuse you're giving it. Your friends don't like it that way. They're getting tired of the abuse you're giving yourself and them too, incidentally. And most of all, *you* don't like it that way. You're tired and worn out from dealing with the problem.

9

It is all going to stop. You are going to stop being what you hate—a fat person who is not in control. Take my hand and let us walk through our lives—step by step. We will learn how to handle people, things and places that we have never before considered problems, or which we have used in ways that are destructive. We're going to take a new look at life. We are going to be kind to ourselves.

Don't race through the program like you used to race through a meal. Stop for a minute and reread this chapter. Put the rules into your head. Make sure that you are ready to take notes. Then step out . . . a person on the way to thinhood. How wonderful! Not a fat person out of control, not a thin person out of control, but simply—a calm person on the way to a good life.

Chapter 11

Being Kind to Yourself

If you are reading this book, then, like me, you've searched everywhere for something to help you end the misery you've been going through for your whole life . . . or the past five years . . . or five months . . . or five days. You also hate yourself for being weak, for having no will power, for not having the strength of your convictions.

That kind of thinking is now over. The only reason you haven't been able to do anything about your weight up until now is that no one ever really told you how. We are now going to learn a totally new way. Don't argue. Don't look for excuses. Listen.

The first thing to understand is that you are a good person. You're not "bad," you're not "weak," you don't have to get up that "will power." The basic thing you have to learn is to be kind to yourself, and most important, that you have a right to a thin life just like everyone else.

You never have to feel deprived again! You are no longer a deprived, anxious, hungry person. You are, from this moment on, one of the fortunates. You are going to learn what it is like to enjoy food, to enjoy your day, to realize accomplishment, to begin each day with renewed hope. You will be able to sit in a restaurant and have everyone envy your lunch and wish they had ordered it. All your friends—including the thin ones—will ask your advice about living a productive life. Because once and for all you're going to find out that you deserve the best. You know that, and together we're going to start an exciting new life, with good health, good friends, good times, and by the way, good food.

Here are some totally new ways of being kind to yourself:

(1) You're going to let everyone around you understand you're living a new life and that they have a role to play in it. I know this is a difficult problem. But it is a solvable one. We'll deal with it over and over again in the book, and you will be able to do it.

(2) You're going to sit down and have a talk with your friends and family about their place in your program. Yes, I know, at least two persons in your home don't have to diet and why should they be deprived? Right? Wrong!

Let's put it this way, and you should tell it to them this way. If you were standing in the middle of your living room on fire, would your nearest and dearest stand around and not help you because *they* weren't on fire? Of course not. Well, you *are* on fire, as sure as if the burning match had been placed at the hem of your skirt or the cuff of your pants. You need everyone's help and cooperation to put out that fire. That means: nothing but what you can eat and what you can deal with can be eaten or can happen in the house *until you can deal with it!* Nothing! One jar of nuts back in the corner for Lucy will form an image in your mind until the moment when you dive into that cupboard and eat every one of those nuts. That's the wrong way to get rid of the wrong things in your house. The right way is with everyone's help and cooperation. If your wife wants pizza, she can have her pizza outside the house, not inside, because . . . YOU ARE BEING KIND TO YOURSELF. If your children want you, their mother, to drive them to the pizzeria, say NO. Say it firmly, say it sweetly, but don't go. BE KIND TO YOURSELF.

(3) You don't go inside any restaurant without knowing in advance what they have on the menu. This way you can be certain that when you order fish, it hasn't been breaded, and you know that they will be happy to broil it for you without butter. How do you know all this? Either because you were there before and you had asked them all these pertinent questions, or because you have called the restaurant yesterday or earlier in the day to ask them. Now you can be certain to have a tasty planned dinner, knowing that eating out can be fun and delicious. You're not deprived, and you're BEING KIND TO YOURSELF.

(4) You don't end this program! You don't have guilt feelings! You don't hate yourself and whip yourself into a frenzy if you eat what you haven't planned. *This is perhaps the most important factor.* The word "cheat" no longer exists in our language. You can call it unplanned eating or whatever you like. It's something that everyone does sometimes . . . and you are no exception. When it happens you must learn to roll with it, and know that when you have finished nothing has happened. You're still on the program, you're certain that your next meal will go as planned. You won't feel guilty. You are a good person who is still in control of your life, still losing weight, and STILL BEING KIND TO YOURSELF.

13

Take a good look at yourself in the mirror. Do it now. Go over there and give it a good once-over. Like that person! That is a good person. That is a person deserving of the best.

My friend Richard, without knowing it, taught me a very important lesson. Richard is thin and has always kept himself in good shape. Like most thin people, he watches his weight. He gets on the scale at least once a week. He looks at himself in the mirror. We joked about this one day and he said, "Look, I want to look the best I can look and feel the best I can feel. It's important to me to know that when I step out the door, I am presenting the best 'Richard' I know how to present. That is why I watch what I eat and why I weigh myself. But more important than that, I want to look good for me. I want to feel good for me. I want to be healthy for me. If I never saw another person again in my whole life, I would still care immensely how I look to myself."

Listen to that sentence. *If I never saw another person again in my whole life, I would still care immensely how I look to myself.* Can you say that about yourself? I must say in all truthfulness that once I couldn't. But that's how I'm feeling about myself now. I'M BEING KIND TO ME . . . I'M TAKING CARE OF ME . . . I'M EATING GOOD FOODS FOR ME . . . AND I'M BECOMING A THIN PERSON FOR ME!

As we move through the book, you will see that the philosophy we are learning together keeps reinforcing this idea.

Of course, in the long run, ending up a thin person is the kindest cut of all. Our goals: to be healthy, to be happy, to be in control of our life, to have renewed hope, to be thin, to be productive. These are all within our grasp simply by our learning HOW TO BE KIND TO OURSELVES.

14

Chapter III

You're Only Human!

At a party the other night my friend Jack told me that the thing that worries him about the program is that it is too demanding. He would have to make too much of a commitment to it. He said, "According to you, I can't ever go to a cocktail party and have an hors d'oeuvre or a drink. I can't see how that could hurt."

Well, it would seem that such a minor indiscretion wouldn't hurt, except that we both have been on diets all our lives. That has been our pattern, and we know what has happened to our diets the moment we began such "minor" indiscretions.

Jack was incensed. He said, "Are you telling me that you are never going to slip? That you are never going to step off the diet once?"

I answered, "Of course I am. The only difference is that *I'm not going to plan it.* Because if I plan it, that will be one time I'm eating foods I shouldn't, and then there will be another time that I eat foods I shouldn't when I *didn't* plan it, and that will make two!"

A couple of weeks ago, I had to go to a meeting in midtown New York, a meeting that was slightly anxiety provoking. When it was over I stopped at a phone booth on the street to call my answering service. I didn't have a dime. I stood on the corner and looked to see where I could get change—a shoe store, a tie store, a furniture store. I walked a little way down Madison Avenue and saw a delicatessen. With my dollar in my hand, I walked straight into the store, stood in line because people were ordering lunches to take out, and when the guy behind the counter looked at me, without a moment's pause I said, "Ham and muenster on a hard roll." He handed me my sandwich and I walked out into the street wondering what in the hell had just happened.

Then I went straight home and ate my sandwich. There's more to say about this incident and others like it, but the point for now is: I had no idea I was going to do this. And if, the night before, when I went to that party, I had allowed myself to eat what I shouldn't, I have no doubt that this would have happened anyway . . . and I would have eaten the wrong things twice in two days instead of once in three weeks.

It is going to happen. We are only human. We are bombarded on all sides by commercials, ads in magazines, signs and smells on the street, food stores everywhere, and by all the years before today when our response to the availability of food was to eat it.

What is our goal here? It is to be in control as much as possible, and when we are out of control, to watch ourselves there, too. To say, when the ham and muenster sandwich is in the mouth, "Look, kid, you're only human.

You're a person who has committed a momentary indiscretion. For a minute those old habits just pushed out from inside you, jumped up over the new ones and made your mouth react like it has for a million years: 'I'll have a ham and muenster on a hard roll, please.' "

This is not being "bad" or "weak" or "slovenly." In fact, face it: we're never going to be completely rid of those familiar patterns, but we're going to try to make the new ones as strong as we can so that such uncontrolled moments happen as rarely as possible. The interesting thing to me is how differently I handled this incident from the way I did my very first indiscretion. As in other life situations, how you handle the first experience is very important to those of the future. Here's what happened the first time:

I had been on the program about six weeks. A friend and I were traveling and dieting together. We had no cooking facilities, so we decided to buy coolers, eat our breakfast and lunch in our rooms and eat our dinners out so that we could practice shopping, preparing food, having food in the room and going to restaurants as well. Everything went perfectly until Joyce told me that she would be visiting relatives for the weekend. This meant that I would be eating dinner Saturday night alone. No problem, I said. Of course I'll be fine. Nothing like eating alone in a small, strange town on a Saturday night, when the person you were supposed to be eating with is having a lovely family dinner. I announced that I would eat at a place that had made us broiled chicken, but I knew in the back of my mind that I was going to head for good ole Colonel Sanders Kentucky Fried. I sat down with my calorie book and rationalized that even if I ate *his* chicken, I could have two pieces and stay within my calories. I had my two beagles with me and decided to get each of them some chicken too, as a treat. Two pieces for each of them and two for me. That's six. I'll order six pieces.

I leapt into my car and drove to the place. With the furtive moves of a bank robber, I parked my car, ran into the Colonel's and looked at all those things all over the wall and then at a list above my right shoulder that contained little extras you can order with your chicken. Biscuits, potatoes, desserts, puddings, hush puppies ... What? "Twelve hush puppies—25 cents." Now, you have to understand what happened here. I was writing down every day the foods that I was eating and the calories they contained. For example:

	Calories
5 ounces chicken	250
cup green beans	30
cup salad	10
apple	80

Well, here I was in Colonel Sanders, and their list looked like this:

	Price
2 biscuits	.25
1 pudding	.40
12 hush puppies	.25

The girl behind the counter said, "Can I help you?," and I said, without blinking or taking a breath, "Yes, six pieces of chicken, which should include two breasts, and twelve hush puppies." There it was, the planned wrong eating (the chicken) and the unplanned happening (the hush puppies) without a moment's pause between them. I didn't even know what hush puppies were! But twelve of them for 25 calories—whoops—25 cents! It took about three minutes for my order to come, and out I ran to the car and put my hands into the mysterious bag. Hush puppies, my dear, are unbelievable—everything a fat person adores, containing everything to keep a fat person fat that one can imagine—little fingers of corn meal loaded with oil and salt. Before three minutes were up I had devoured all twelve of those buggers and was stuffed. Started up the car and drove back to the motel, cleaned the chicken off the bone for my dogs and ate my own chicken in about two seconds—with excruciating anxiety and breathlessness.

It was done. I sat there practically panting, when the most compelling thirst welled up inside me. You see, I had been salt-free for six weeks and never felt thirsty. Now all I could think of was Tab, Diet-Rite, cola. I also wanted to eat more. It was as though I had unleashed a wellspring of desire. I wanted to stay in control but I felt so damn guilty for having eaten what I had eaten, I felt such pain and anxiety that I decided that I had to have Shasta Diet Chocolate. After several phone calls to supermarkets, I finally found one that carried Shasta and drove there instantly. I walked straight to the diet soda counter, bought four bottles, and started to walk out of the store. But of course, the diet foods were placed directly next to the bakery department. I tried to walk past the department, but my legs were riveted to the floor. I was standing in front of a display counter that had what looked like homemade layer cakes cut in half. These had to be the highest layer cakes ever made in the history of the world, eighteen layers at least. The ingredients were listed on the outside of the clear plastic wrap. I picked up each of those cakes and read all those unbelievable ingredients to myself. Walnuts, coconut, pecans, diamonds, richness, stocks, bonds, marriage . . . Don't ask me how I got out of that store alive. But I did. I read the ingredients on every cake, held every one in my hand, and walked to the checkout counter with my four bottles of diet soda. Got in my car and back to the motel—and drank myself sick. Sick and full, I finally fell asleep. The next morning I weighed myself. I had gained four pounds. It took me a week to get back to the weight I was that Saturday.

Now, the difference between this time and the "Madison Avenue incident." Then I took my sandwich home. I was calm. I told myself that I was only human and was just behaving like my old self—except that the old self was fat and the new self was not and was not ever going to be again. I would eat this sandwich calmly, enjoying it and knowing that when I finished it, I was still on my program. Nothing had happened but a slight jog on my straight and narrow path. I would keep it in its proper perspective—no guilt. I hadn't done wrong. I was not bad. I was not weak. I was a person with a momentary indiscretion. I was a person on her way to thinhood. The lack of guilt allowed me to put the brake on this moment of unplanned eating. Combine guilt and anxiety with unplanned eating and you've got a food orgy. We're never going to have to deal with that again. You're a person, you're a good person, but you're only human—the important thing is that *you are in control,* and that makes everything possible.

Chapter IV

The Support System: You Don't Do This on Your Own

You are not alone when you are on this program. All the items listed below are there to help you, to give you something to lean on, something you can count on. With each of these in your life, every minute of your day can be controlled, by you, without pain and effort.

Don't forget, anyone who has ever tried to get life control knows exactly how you feel. I've been there. I'm there now. Together we're going to climb the mountain.

Each time you use any of the items in the support system, you are unconsciously reminding yourself that you are indeed on the program. They will help keep you in line. Each of them performs an important function in keeping you and your program working and moving ahead.

Here are the elements of the support system:

(1) The scale
(2) The diary

(3) The calorie book
(4) Measuring implements
(5) Measuring yourself
(6) The doctor
(7) Structuring your time
(8) The miracle exercise
(9) The graph of success

The scale

Take a stand and weigh in!

If you don't already have one, you're buying a scale for *YOU* because *YOU MATTER.* You're even going to go out and buy the one that you really like, not the one that's the cheapest, because you deserve to do good things for yourself. You deserve the best.

A scale used to be a negative idea—the ugly, mechanical device that showed you that you were out of control. Now it is something that will show you that you are in control of your life. Every day will be another measure of the success you're going to attain.

If you or any of us could afford it, the scale in the doctor's office is the one to have. You can really read 1/4-ounce gains and losses, and it is really accurate. Unfortunately, those scales are extraordinarily expensive. However, there are some smaller versions of that stand-up scale available in discount stores and chains. They are not totally out of the question and are indeed more accurate than most.

But the truth is it doesn't matter. It only matters that YOU have a scale that you weigh yourself on every morning before you eat and before you get dressed, and that you keep weighing yourself on your own scale.

Getting on the scale in the morning should become as automatic as getting dressed, a part of your life pattern. You are, after all, measuring your body in relation to your life. In my mind, the weight of my body is completely responsible for what I feel I deserve and what I will allow myself to get from life—or what I will allow myself to give to life. If you are like me, we're not just weighing pounds here, we're weighing life. Instantly every morning, you're going to know where you are.

Write down in your diary (we're discussing that next) your weight today and every day. We will also discuss your relationship with your doctor in a later chapter, and you can be weighed in that office too. It's fun to keep a record of what you weigh in a different place, because as sure as shootin' the scales will differ.

We lose weight in a complicated way which is a very individual thing. After you keep track of your weight for a while, you will start to notice a pattern. It could be like this: Monday –1/4 lb.; Tuesday –1/4 lb.; Wednesday 0; Thursday 0; Friday –1 3/4 lbs.; Saturday +1/4 lb.; Sunday 0.

A person with a pattern like this will lose a little, then the scale won't change. Then there will be a big loss, then probably a weight gain and again a no-change. This is a typical loss pattern and is, as you can see, very erratic. Also bear in mind that the minor fluctuations, a quarter pound here and there, don't count. It's the daily support of stepping on the scale that's important.

I think we should also spend a little time talking about the most perplexing problem of them all—*the plateau.* This is when, even though you are perfectly in control of your program, the scale does not budge. You neither lose nor gain, or you lose a quarter pound one day and gain it back the next. This can be very discouraging, but you must hold on. The weight is being lost. As a matter of fact, when you are measuring yourself (see page 36) you will see changes. But the losses just aren't being reflected on the scale. It is a common problem, and when it happens to you, whether it's three days or three weeks, be assured that you are doing nothing wrong. If you stick with the program, the losses will begin again.

The diary

Keeping a diary is a good healthy idea, a wonderful way to keep in touch with our feelings, to keep in touch with our life. We all have a tendency to hide from ourselves how we really feel. Maybe that's one of the reasons our weight got out of control.

We're going to incorporate the diary into our lives. It will perform amazing functions. We will be writing down our daily feelings and experiences, and it will therefore eventually become a history of our life.

We'll be able to look back and see if we can tell who or what helped us to stay in control. Were we always out of control when we ate dinner alone? Or after a large weight loss? The wonderful part about all of this is that we don't have to ask ourselves *why* we react in this way to these situations or persons—only *if* we do. If we see something happening with a regular pattern, we can do something about it. If your diary reveals that each time you're with your friend Alice, she says something like "Why are you eating that? I thought you were on a diet," and you react by continuing to eat something fattening, you have at least two choices of how to deal with the situation. You could, once and for all, tell Alice not to say those things because they hurt your feelings and are counterproductive, that you would rather she never again mentioned your diet, that you don't need a policeman. If you did, you'd hire one, right? Or if for some reason you can't do that or she can't understand, then perhaps you will decide to start seeing less of Alice. That's really possible, you know. No one needs to have a thorn in their side. The healthy thing—but sometimes the hardest—is to pull out the thorn. It may hurt more for a moment, but afterward the relief more than makes up for it.

So write down the whole experience—that's what the diary is all about. It's you and it's yours alone. There are not enough things in your life that belong just to you.

Go to the store and touch and look at all the available diaries. Take one that feels as if it belongs in *your* hand. Then put it by your bed, or in your pocket. It's like the log the captain of a ship keeps, or the pilot of a plane. It serves two purposes: it's a plan that sets the goals for the day; then it becomes a record of what really happened that day.

There is a sample diary at the back of the book and, as you can see, it records what you're going to eat today, including the calories, as well as what you intend to do with your time.

Just as important, at the end of the day, write down exactly what you did eat, if you didn't eat exactly what you planned. Write exactly what you did do, if you didn't do what you had planned—and exactly how you felt either during the day or later when you were looking back.

The diary is another tool to remind ourselves that we are on the program, another click in our brain to keep us on the path. It is so easy to stop weighing ourselves, stop writing in the diary and stop being on the program, but somehow, when *all* the systems are working, we are re-minded of what our job is, and it is easier to stay in control.

Use the diary in this book. Begin today. Using this one at first will keep you close to the book, and for a while that's important. Because this book should be another one of your support systems. Keep it beside you. Reread chapters. Read the chapter that pertains to what you're doing as you're doing it. Going to the supermarket? Read that chapter again today.

How to use it:

First thing every morning, weigh yourself and write your weight in your diary. Make sure your meals are planned for the day. You will see how to do this on page 60. Your meal plan is in your diary. Now write down the day's activities. If you work, most of that time is taken care of. But if you don't go out to work or if it's the weekend, then a whole empty day faces you. Let's talk about this full empty day first.

What do you *plan* to do today? If you see from your diary that there are blocks of time with nothing sched-uled, plan them now. Don't leave yourself with empty periods of time. TIME ON YOUR HANDS IS FOOD IN YOUR MOUTH! Invite someone over, invite yourself to some-one's house. Go to a movie, to the library, to the gym to work out. Go shopping, do that sewing you've been put-ting off, take your pants to the tailor's. Write the letters you always mean to write. Take a well-deserved nap, go to a concert, take a lovely long walk. You will be amazed at how much can be accomplished in a day that is planned versus a day that is not planned.

If you work during the day, make certain that your evening is taken care of. Don't find yourself sitting alone in front of the television with a refrigerator waiting for you. Plan activities like those we've just talked about for "during the day." Think of all the things you seem to never have time to do, things that you keep putting off. Now is the time to do them. Use your diary to spot the trouble periods and to plan for them. You are going to find that time is opening up for you. With less emphasis on food, it seems we've added hours to our day. We've added life to our life.

Now, write down how you felt yesterday. If you had uncontrolled eating yesterday, see if you can detect why. Was it because you caught a glimpse of yourself in a store window, and you don't yet look like the person you want to be? Was it because you tried on clothes, and you're not yet the size you want to be? Try to find out what things set you off. If you can detect a pattern, you may be able to avoid the very thing that makes you have moments of uncontrolled eating. The more we know about the times when we are out of control, the more those moments come under our control.

You may also find other patterns of moods. For example, some women find that a few days prior to their menstruation they have feelings of anxiety which can be translated into a need to eat or a need for sugar. Keep track of your menstrual period in the diary too, and see if you notice any pattern here.

If you seem to be eating more before your period, realize where those feelings are coming from and make an extra effort to stay in control. The diary will help you beat another old habit!

Male or female, we all have mood cycles. The diary will help us to recognize them. Some are physiological, and some are caused by very specific happenings in our lives. Perhaps when we are traveling out of town on business and find ourselves without company at mealtimes, hating the loneliness of the hotel room, *boom,* food enters our mind. If that's happening to you, think hard. There are ways to fill those empty times. Call an old friend you haven't looked up in years. Plan some writing—maybe that novel you've always wanted to try or letters you always wanted to write. Maybe it's time to really get into Marx (Groucho or the other one). Maybe it's time to reread *anything* by Dickens. The secret is to plan it in advance, write it in your diary, and the next thing you know—you're doing it!

It is important to say here that more times than not, you are entitled to feel what you feel. As you reread the record, you may start to notice that every time your in-laws are coming to dinner, you eat your way through the night after they have gone home. Or every time you have a confrontation with your boss about money may be when you eat. Knowing it, can stave it off. Don't judge yourself. Don't tell yourself you shouldn't feel the way you feel. Allow yourself to feel everything. The point is: don't use your feelings as an excuse to eat. Eating your way through the refrigerator solves nothing. It only calms you for a moment, and then you start feeling guilty, anxious—and eating ensues again. Don't let food be the punctuation for every moment of feeling in your life. FEEL, KNOW YOU'RE ALIVE—AND IN CONTROL!

As to *uncontrolled* eating . . . write it down when it occurs. That's not a punishment, it's something to learn from. What did you choose to eat? When did you eat it? Why did you eat one particular thing rather than another? How many calories was it? How did you come out for the day? Sometimes the thought of the uncontrolled eating is worse than the reality. If you ate the whole potato instead of cutting it in half, it may only have been 45 extra calories that you took in for the day. That is still a victory. But the guilt you may feel over eating the whole potato can turn the thing into a disastrous moment and keep you off the straight and narrow. Don't lie to *you.* Tell it all . . . that's what the diary is for.

Remember, you are the most important person in the world to you, and you want to be thin. Wanting it enough is what's going to make it happen.

The calorie book

(Buy two—one for using and one for losing.)

"Outwitting ourselves" is what we should be calling this section. This can be wonderful fun. A calorie book is like uncovering the secrets of the stars. We really need to understand the amazing differences in caloric content in food to see how we can eat better and even "more" by watching where we put our calories.

To shop for "your" calorie book, go to the best book store in town. Take with you a sample menu or a list of some favorite foods that you wish could be on the program. Look through each book and find specific items. See which book works best for you. Try to incorporate one of the invaluable brand-name calorie books in your choice. After you've found the book that is right for you, buy three—one for the kitchen, one for your pocket and one for losing.

Play a game with me. Choose 100 calories and see what you can get in the righthand column versus what you're not going to eat, and probably think you want to eat, on the left.

	Not Eating	Eating

Not Eating	Eating
(Each item has 100 calories)	
20 peanuts	1 1-pound lobster
2 slices of bacon	2 cups of bean sprouts
1 tablespoon of butter	1 whole canteloupe
1 Coke	3 cups of cauliflower
2 cookies	3 ounces of tuna fish
1 tablespoon mayonnaise	6 egg whites
1 tablespoon peanut butter	4 1/2 ounces of haddock
9 potato chips	2 1/2 cups of mushrooms
1 ounce of steak	1 whole baked potato
3/4 cup of winter squash	3 1/2 cups of summer squash
1 medium banana	30 strawberries
1/2 waffle	2 ounces of bran flakes

Amazing, huh! Do you know how long it would take me to polish off twenty peanuts? Right. We're both experts at it. But to eat and enjoy a lobster, to do it right, I'd say would take me an hour. I'll take the lobster every time and so will you.

Play the game, you'll enjoy it. You'll also find out that it's one of the most important games of your life. There is a real concept to be found here. It's called "paying attention."

Too much of what we do wrong we do just because it's a habit. Breakfast may just mean a glass of orange juice. But when you realize that it can take up almost all of your calories and contains no protein, you start rethinking your priorities.

You always put butter on your baked potatoes, so if you're going on a diet, you can't have that potato any more. WRONG. Enjoy the potato. It's only 90 to 100 calories, and it doesn't need butter to be delicious. My own rule is baked potato only with fish and at least two vegetables with chicken. Here are two sample meals:

The New Way		The Old Way	
7 ounces of striped bass	210	7 ounces of striped bass cooked in butter	310
1 cup of Brussels sprouts	50	1 cup of Brussels sprouts with 2 teaspoons of butter	110
1 baked potato	100	1 baked potato with 1 tablespoon of sour cream	200
1 portion of salad	10	1 portion of salad	10
1 tablespoon of low-calorie dressing	6	1 tablespoon of regular dressing	75
1/4 canteloupe	25	1/4 canteloupe	25
total	401	total	730

The second meal tastes no better than the first. But in the second meal, almost twice as many calories have been consumed.

I like to think what an exciting time this is for those of us who are smart enough to know that counting calories is the only way to be in control of a diet program. Luckily, every product in the supermarket soon will be marked with the calorie content clearly in view.

There are three calorie books that I use, listed below, but you should use whatever book seems easiest for you.

The All-in-One Calorie Counter by Jean Carper; Bantam, $1.50.

The Brand Name Nutrition Counter by Jean Carper; Bantam, $1.95.

The Basic Food & Brand-Name Calorie Counter by Barbara Kraus; Grosset & Dunlap, $1.50.

Don't guess at anything. Look it up. Figure it out. If you decide to make a big stew that requires a million ingredients—carrots, celery, tomatoes—write down each item beforehand. Figure out the calorie content. Figure out how many cups you are making and know exactly how many calories you are taking in when you eat a cup measure of it. Nothing is free. On this program there is no such thing as eating as much of anything as you want. First of all, we don't need to be eating at all hours of the day and night. We only eat three meals a day. Three delicious meals a day. Three calorie-counted meals a day. We know where we are, exactly how many calories we have consumed and how many are left to be consumed at any given moment of the day. The calorie book is very much like the scale. It doesn't matter which one you use. Just keep using the same one, because calorie counts do vary from book to book. I suppose accurate information is hard to get, and definition sometimes gets in the way.

The place where I have found the most discrepancy is with fish, raw or cooked. What I have finally determined for myself is that nonfatty fishes such as sole, flounder, haddock and cod are all about 20 calories per ounce raw. When the fish is cooked, the calories change because of shrinkage. I count approximately 30 calories per ounce for cooked fish, whether it is broiled, poached, baked or boiled. For fatty fishes such as salmon, halibut and turbot, you've got to figure about 50 calories an ounce cooked.

A calorie book will enable you to understand and appreciate the uniqueness of foods as well. I never gave much thought to squash, and thought all squash was the same. Of course, they're not. They don't taste the same, and the calories are extraordinarily different. Summer squashes, the crookneck and zucchini, are very low in calories, 25 to 30 calories a cup. Winter squashes, acorn and butternut, are about 70 to 100 calories a cup. Of course, you may find that a half a cup of the winter squash is quite sufficient, compared to a whole cup of summer squash.

Keep your calorie book beside you when you sit down to plan your meals for the week. Look up every item until it becomes second nature to you. Learn to see by size and quantity how much a cup of cauliflower is, how large a 100-calorie potato is as compared to a 200-calorie potato (a 6-ounce raw potato is approximately 90 to 100 calories). Then when you go out to eat and can't weigh things, and you have to know how much to eat of what you're given, you'll be able to recognize the proper quantity.

Take your calorie book with you to the supermarket. The brand-name calorie books are especially helpful. I know that you will be shopping with a preprepared shopping list, but sometimes you will happen upon a new vegetable or a new packaged frozen vegetable—and you ought to be able to know how many calories are in it before you consider buying it.

Take your calorie book with you when you go out to eat. Sometimes, even if you prepare for your meal out, things can happen that are potential disasters. They could be out of baked potatoes or vegetables, or you may have been given misinformation and they only cook their vegetables with butter, so you can't have them. Therefore, you may determine to make a substitution in what you have planned. Pull out the calorie book and consult.

Take the calorie book with you when you go to a friend's house for a meal. As much as you may try to be in control of what you're eating, it is always harder when you are in someone else's house. Your host may play switchee with you and think it doesn't matter. Just pull out your calorie book and make a determination. After all, they may think fish means any kind of fish. You have allotted yourself so many calories for a low-calorie fish and they surprise you proudly with abalone. Look it up. Yes, sir, it's one of the lean fishes: 3½ ounces, raw, 98 calories. But it could have been pompano: yipes! 4 ounces, 188 calories. Keep that little book beside you. It will help to keep you in control and out of trouble.

Measuring implements

Everything measured—nothing gained!

In a completely confused world, it is very reassuring to know that measuring implements exist and we don't have to go around guessing. Because you have measured every inch of it, you can be quite sure that when you sit down to eat that wonderful bowl of cereal, cottage cheese and peaches for breakfast, 150 calories is exactly what you are eating. No more, no less, and—hooray—you are entitled to every ounce of it!

Here's what you need:

A kitchen scale

Again, any one will do, versus none. I prefer a scale that has some kind of dish or platform to measure into. Your scale should go to a minimum of 16 ounces, and if possible, to 2 or 3 pounds. You will find that when you want to weigh raw fish, for example, more than a one-pound scale is often necessary. If you don't have a scale with this weight, have your butcher or fish person weigh it for you in the store, and write it on the package. Get a scale with the dial large enough to read. I don't think a postage scale is sufficient, but it's better than nothing.

If you eat cereal, every morning you should measure it out onto your scale. One ounce of bran buds is quite different from one ounce of raisin bran or one ounce of puffed wheat. You will be amazed.

Measuring scoops

Half-cup, 1/3-cup, 1/4-cup and 2-tablespoon measuring scoops are invaluable. Even though you measure out 1/4 cup of cottage cheese every day, and think you should know by now exactly what 1/4 cup is, still, with the scoop, you know you have exactly the right amount, and haven't picked up an inflated concept over a period of time.

Measuring spoons

Probably you already have these in your house for cooking. Keep them handy on your counter so that they are always right there when you need them.

Measuring cups

Get a 1-cup, 2-cup and 3-cup measure, all in Pyrex so that you can measure hot things right off the stove. For serving, instead of a large spoon, use a measuring cup. It accomplishes the same purpose and *voilà!* If you're to have a cup of cooked cauliflower, in one twist of the wrist, you have measured it directly from the stove onto your plate.

I find that I really enjoy taking the time to measure things out and use each of my implements. Maybe I am finally living out the fantasy of being in one of those old B-movies where mad scientists stood in their laboratories, with cauldrons boiling, and poured mysterious liquids from one test tube to another.

Well, Dr. Thin Person, measure away. Enjoy every minute of it. Each moment of measuring reassures you again that you are in control here. This is your life and you're going to make the most of it—even if the most is exactly "one cup," or "4 ounces" or "a pinch"!

Measuring yourself

See yourself as others see you!

When you're on a weight-losing program the inches are going to change. Sometimes they're not visible to the eye, but the trusty old tape measure knows the truth and tells all. Each time that measure tells you you're a smaller person is equivalent to receiving the Academy Award. Imagine receiving such kudos every week.

When you start this program you will need everything available to keep you going. Measuring yourself is an invaluable support. It is so specific, so absolute—because you just can't discount numbers. There it is, in black and white, proof that your program is working, that you are learning to be in control of your life, that you are on your way to being a thin person.

Buy a cheap tape measure in the five-and-ten—not a metal one, but the kind that has big clear numbers on fabric or plastic.

Now take a page in your diary, or if you enjoy making up charts, make a big one and attach it to the door of your refrigerator or closet or bathroom. Use different colors. For example:

Part of Body	Measurement					
				Month		
Week	7	14	21	28	5	1 2
Neck						
Upper arm						
Forearm						
Wrist						
Finger						
Bust						
Chest						
Area above the waist						
Waistline						
Abdomen						
Hips						
Upper thigh						
Calf						
Ankle						
Width of foot						

As painful as it may be when you start, measure your-self from the beginning of the program—because the payoff is so fantastic! Set a particular day and time in the week when you are going to measure yourself, and mea-sure in the same position each time. For example, when you have to bend over to measure your legs, their size changes. Your figures for your upper thigh are going to be different when you do it yourself from what they are when you stand upright and someone else measures you.

No matter what kind of tape measure you use, no matter where you write it down and how you take the measurements—you are going to find that this is not a trivial task. It is another important cog in the total support system you are setting up to help yourself stay on the program.

Even when the scale doesn't move, sometimes for one, two or three weeks, as we were discussing earlier, if you're measuring yourself and keeping a chart, you'll see that the inches are indeed changing.

For those of you who have relatively little to lose, with just the right amount of dieting your weight may hardly change, but you'll see the inches move around, and soon you will appear thinner.

We should also deal here with something that may be very frustrating to you. WE LOSE LAST WHERE WE NEED IT MOST! I don't know why—maybe because that's the first place we put it on. You've seen how some people with large hips start to get very thin in the face and waist before it really starts to happen where it counts. "However you lose it . . . measure it.!"

The miracle excercise

If you hate to exercise, you'll love this section!

Walking every day, in addition to keeping to a good solid food program, can make all the difference in how much you lose, how fast you lose, where you lose and how your body tone will be after you've lost the weight.

Walking is the miracle exercise.

I know! I know! The word exercise is enough to keep

many of you from even reading this chapter. But this program has nothing to do with the "lift your arm," "lower your body" routine.

We've just finished talking about structuring your day. All you have to do now is write into your schedule: "Take a walk."

Walking is one of the few exercises that almost everyone can do. The kind of walking we're talking about is just like ordinary walking—except that you are going to concentrate on it a little.

The best way is to have planned at least a half-hour of uninterrupted walking, a walk for a walk's sake. Go around your neighborhood, circle the shopping plaza, walk to the station, walk home from work, walk up and down your hall.

First: plan the time. Second: try to walk unencumbered. If you can possibly manage it, carry no pocketbooks or brief cases, nothing in your hands, wear no tight underclothes, no constricting ties or collars. Until you do it, you will never understand how terrific it is to begin that brisk walk. Let your arms swing in the air, and feel your entire body responding to the rhythm of your walk.

I remember when I first started to "walk." It was only a year ago, and I began after I noticed how everybody's rear end was undulating. Hips were moving, arms swinging. Then I compared it to my walk and realized that, with me, nothing was moving. I was tight as a new shoe. I then realized that because over the years I had gotten so fat, I had deliberately forced myself to walk as rigidly as possible so that the fat wouldn't move around and I wouldn't look . . . God knows what I hoped I wouldn't look like.

If this strikes a familiar chord, work on it. Walk with your hands on your hips so that you can feel them start moving. Try to feel something happening with your waist. Even if that part of your anatomy is hard to find —inside, there is one. If you use that area a bit when you walk, you may find it.

Soon your body will get the idea, and you will feel like a new person. The half of you that hasn't moved in years will get mobility, and the more it moves, the more energy you have.

See if you can do your regular distance faster tomorrow than today. Can you increase how far you walk and do it in the same amount of time? Of course you can, and you will. At the beginning set a goal for yourself of a one-mile walk, twice a day. Then make it a two-mile walk twice a day. It doesn't matter when, but plan it. Write it into your diary. Know in the morning when you're going to do it.

The idea of this program is that we're being kind to ourselves. Well, you can't do that if your feet hurt. Try on every walking shoe made until you find the one which makes you feel you don't have a shoe on your foot. You may have to go to a sports store to find it. You may discover that one of the official jogging or walking shoes is right, or the old-fashioned saddle, or the new-fangled crepe soles. Find your shoe, put it on with socks or stockings or whatever is most comfortable. (Forget about how things look—we're only interested in comfort now. Remember: we're only to be concerned about ourselves, no one else.)

As to clothes, wear what makes you comfortable: a jogging suit? Fine. Shorts and a T-shirt? Terrific. Slacks and a sweat shirt? Great. Pick clothes that let you move and don't inhibit you, that tell you that you're out for the walk and for nothing else at that moment.

We're talking now about walking under optimum conditions, but I don't mean to negate the walk to the office, or the one you do while you're shopping. They all count.

They all mean you're moving, you're filling your time, you're exercising your body. Specific walks, though, work more efficiently.

What does the walking do? Besides making us know that we are alive, while we're losing weight walking keeps everything tightening, keeps your skin texture healthy. When people lose large amounts of weight, there is often a rather slack look to the skin. If you walk, your skin will hold its elasticity and look tight and healthy.

Of course, walking is also burning up calories—how many is not important. But you don't have to look for a reason to do it. Rather, the concept of the "good walk" will become a part of your life habit because you enjoy it. It will be something you do every day, just as you eat three meals a day.

Certainly, swimming, jogging, running, bike riding, jumping rope are all terrific ways to exercise. An exercycle lets you get really good exercise when the weather is bad. But use caution with all of these activities if you are more than a little overweight. Talk to your doctor about it because your weight, age, health, all have to be taken into consideration.

I remember a terrific precautionary measure given by the track coach at Duke: no matter what the exercise, every few minutes say a sentence out loud. If you find that you can't talk above a whisper without gasping for breath, then stop and rest. No exercise, including walking, should ever make you unable to speak a sentence.

What is the brain doing while the body is busy with that walk? The brain, my dears, literally eats up this time. It works out problems, gets rid of anxieties and begins perceiving life with a sparkling clarity you have not known in ages. Walking really gives your head a chance to sort things out.

41

You know, we are so lucky to only be fat—because we can get thin. Think of all those people who have things wrong with them that they can't do anything about. We're already on the way to getting rid of our problem, and we're doing it by being good to ourselves. By such beautiful activities as walking.

Let's repeat.

(1) Plan your walking in the morning. Write it in your diary: when, where and with whom, if anybody.

(2) Walk unencumbered.

(3) Let the whole body swing free. Make it all move!

(4) Get some good walking shoes.

Take a well-earned rest

Walk into your bedroom, pull down the shades, turn off the television, the radio. Take off your clothes. Lie down on your cool bed, let your head rest on the soft pillowcase —and rest. Let all thoughts leave your head, all problems.

Look, what have you got to think about? You've planned your day. A rest is part of your plan; you're just fulfilling a planned activity.

You need this time, no matter who you are, what you do—whether you're a housewife, accountant, busy executive, harassed student. There is time in your life for a rest, every day.

You don't have to sleep, but you shouldn't fight it either. Give yourself about half an hour to an hour, and then get up and go on to the next planned activity. Stop for one second and notice: you never felt better in your life. You deserve such good times. No one ever deserved them more!

Structuring your time

The most important thing I can warn you about is: TIME ON YOUR HANDS IS FOOD IN YOUR MOUTH!

You must plan your day, each hour, if necessary, with as much care and concern as you plan your food. Look at your life. Think about when the bad times are for you and food, and you will see how often such times occur because you decided to cancel whatever it was you had planned to do—so you could stay home and "take it easy for a change."

The bad time for many people with a "nine-to-five" job is Saturday. They work so hard all week that when it comes to Saturday they make no plans. They want to stay home, put their feet up and watch an old movie on television.

Fine. Except that when you do those things, you eat. There is no miracle formula that will allow you to sit around all day in your house and not eat the food in the refrigerator. Indeed, that will probably be all you will be thinking about.

You yourself may have structured your bad times right into your life. One woman I know worked, by her own choice, until three o'clock in the afternoon. It was something she had planned when her children were younger. Now her children were in college, but she still came home at three o'clock. And she realized that the period between three and five in the afternoon was a total eating disaster for her.

The solution is simple. She should extend her job to five o'clock, or make plans to take a class at three o'clock. Make outside appointments at three, go to the library at three. Do anything, but don't just "go home." By continuing this pattern, she would continue to have the bad time

43

and never be able to resist the food around her.

I don't mean to demean the excuses we all think up. They seem perfectly sensible to us, but telling them to others makes them seem silly and lame.

Making excuses is behaving as though we are victims. WE ARE NOT VICTIMS. We can be in control of our lives. We can use our time joyously and productively. Thinking about food wastes our lives. THE MORE YOU DO, THE MORE ENERGY YOU HAVE TO DO MORE! Think about the most productive times in your life. They were always times that were too busy. But you felt alive and your thoughts were alive. Not only were you productive for others, you were extraordinarily productive for yourself.

Think, first of all, about the time during the day that is hardest for you to handle food. Figure out how this period can be changed, not *why* you can't handle it. "Handling" is that old barbarian concept of "Be strong," "Use a little will power," "You're behaving like a child." Forget all that. We're trying to make life easier for ourselves, to be kind to ourselves. We're going to change the bad periods of the day to good ones by restructuring our time. We're going to live beautifully. And the kindest thing you can do for yourself is to insert in that bad time of day a new thing, something that can give you more pleasure than eating, preferably something that will bring you in contact with people. Think it over: you will come up with a realistic, happy solution.

Whether you're dealing with the hard times in the daytime or in the evening, depending on whether you're at home or you're working, you can enroll in a class, form a regular card game, consider a part-time job, a game of squash, a regular walk with a friend—but something you can plan and count on.

After you've dealt with the hard part, the rest of the

day will fall into place. Sit down with your diary in the morning and fill in the day's activities first before you even think about the food.

Fill in the hours. Even if it seems silly to write down "car pool" or "work" or "movie" or "resting"—write them all down.

When you do this, you're protecting yourself. You're removing the pitfalls, picking up all the banana peels in advance instead of pretending you don't see them.

Every day we'll cope only with today. That's enough for one day.

WE ARE NOT VICTIMS. WE ARE IN CONTROL OF OUR LIVES. WE ARE PEOPLE WITH HOPE. WE WILL PLAN OUR DAY AND PROTECT OURSELVES FROM PAIN!

TIME ON OUR HANDS IS FOOD IN OUR MOUTHS!

Sharing it with your doctor

There are doctors who push varicolored pills or who play shoot-'em-up or who experiment with your life as they plan another best-selling fad diet. Forget them. We are talking about support systems here. We're not really looking for a doctor who's going to help us diet, although a few of them have studied nutrition and behavior and know something about the problem.

If the doctor is worth anything, your health is his first concern, and he will be in favor of this program. He may not know how to implement it, but he will know how to support it. This is what you want.

Check in, explain the program, and if you haven't done so recently, have a complete physical. You don't *have* to do this, but the results of this program are so spectacular that it will be fun to see them verified scientifically. There will be changes in your measurements, your blood pressure, your sugar count and your cholesterol level. There will be real physical evidence that you're a success story.

After the initial examination, check in to the doctor once a month, just to be weighed and have your blood pressure taken. Make arrangements with the doctor's nurse to sneak in before or after the rush. Have her keep a chart on you, and mark the figures down on your own chart at home. You can be in and out in three minutes. Most good physicians will be so thrilled you're doing something good for yourself, and that you are doing it so intelligently, that they will be more than willing to cooperate.

Even after you're a thin person, on maintenance, a regular check-up will serve as another reminder that you are still on your program.

Use the doctor as a sounding board if you can. Depending on your relationship and how much support you can count on, your doctor is a terrific person to talk to when you feel that you need some help in getting over the rough times. Make sure you've shown the doctor this book and that you've clearly explained the program. Then when you're sure of his understanding, ask if you may call when necessary for his support. I think you'll find again that he is eager to help.

Chapter V

How to Deal with Your Family While You're Getting Thin

"How can I possibly get rid of all the fattening things in the house? My husband is a thin person, and he needs his bread and cookies and candies!"

"My wife loves to cook and give fancy gourmet dinner parties. How can I deprive her of pleasure just because I have to get rid of these extra pounds?"

Sound familiar? For every fat person in the world, or for every person who needs to lose weight, there's someone very near by who never gains a pound, no matter what he eats. Right? Wrong!

If you paid attention you would see that the thin person eats less. How many times have you seen that thin person leave half a piece of pie? My God, how can anyone do that? I can't even imagine it. But thin people do indeed do that. You perceive only that they are eating pie. The fact of the matter is that most of the time they don't eat much of what you think they're eating. *Nobody stays thin by eating as much as you think they eat.*

It's very difficult to issue ultimatums to people who don't have to watch their weight just because *you* do have to watch yours. But you must remember: they care about you and want to help you. Probably they just don't know how.

Us food-o-holics are secretive and shy about discussing our food passions and desires with those closest to us. The first step in doing away with this destructive behavior is to tell ourselves, "Look, I know I'm out of control. It's nothing to be ashamed of. I've got a problem that's got to be licked, and I don't have to be doing it by myself. Let me enlist the aid of those around me who care. Perhaps if I tell them the truth about my compulsiveness, they may not be appalled—they may understand. They may have something just like it in their own lives."

I remember my friend Win telling about the time he ate approximately fourteen pounds of pistachio nuts, just sitting at home alone one night with this unbelievable bowl in front of him and shelling and eating those pistachios as fast as he could. Worrying should he open a dozen and then eat all twelve of them at once, or open each separately so that they would be in his mouth faster. He did both, alternating, depending on his mood. Now twelve, now one. Finding himself, as he ate more and more, becoming more intensely involved with the mechanics of it, opening one pistachio shell by using another as a wedge, finding the right rhythm, finding time becoming a blur. The only thing that was important was getting those nuts into his mouth. Several hours later he found himself limp and satiated and all fourteen pounds of pistachios gone. The mountain of shells piled up in front of him was a brutal reminder of a time of complete madness.

And Win is a thin person. Someone very much in control. After telling us this hysterical, mad story, he told us that there is one area where he still has a constant problem: Peanut Butter Cups. Traveling out of town a lot, he would often stop by the newsstand in his hotel to pick up the paper before he went to his room for the night. Paying for the paper, he would glance down at the candy stand and always find staring at him . . . the Peanut Butter Cups. With one continuous motion, he would pick them up and wave them at the newsstand person without missing a beat. The money for the paper and the cups would be taken out of his dollar, and off he would go to his room. He would do all his nighttime ablutions, get into bed, open the paper, open the Peanut Butter Cups and, in one second, he would have devoured them. Then he'd find himself putting his pants back on, his shoes (no socks), his coat, and making his way out the door, down in the elevator (twenty floors, thirty floors—what did it matter?), across the lobby, over to the newsstand, two-three-four-five-six packages of Cups, no paper as a ruse, staring at the newsdealer and saying to himself, "You betcha, fella, I want all six of these. Just take the money—no wisecracks." Clutching them in his hand, he'd make his way back up to his room and devour them.

Win can't believe that anything would have made him get up out of his bed as tired as he was, as late as it was, but something did. He has just had to eliminate that something from his life. He can't handle those candies, he can't handle one. And therefore he does not allow himself to have even one.

It's hilarious, but it's terrifying, too. It's exactly like the alcoholic who is not able to handle one drink. The important thing is to recognize the problem and then do anything to spare yourself the agony. Don't think that you're weak if you can't eat just one. You're like a lot of people, but if they are thin they have probably eliminated that particular madness from their lives.

The real difference between you and the thin person is that most of the time you succumb and sometimes you are in control . . . Most of the time thin people are in control and sometimes they succumb. You just have to change that formula around and you'll be a thin person, too.

A woman I'll call Harriet lives in Cleveland, and her story is a classic in the behavior of husbands and wives when one of the partners is overweight. Harriet's husband Tom was told by his doctor that he needed to lose a lot of weight. Harriet and I talked about how they were going to handle it. I asked her, "What does he eat that makes him put on weight? "Bread," she said. "Bread, bagels— and a lot of nighttime eating after I've gone to bed." I said, "Well, you'll stop bringing bagels and bread into the house, right?" *Silence.* And I notice that her eyes are showing fury. Finally she hit out, "Tom doesn't need me to do anything. When he makes up his mind to lose weight, he always does it. All anyone needs is will power, and he's got it. I should know, because he's done this a million times before." I explained that at this time in his life Tom can't afford to lose those fifty pounds and then put them on again. It's not will power we're talking about. We're talking about a new way of life they've got to share together.

Back came Harriet: "Well, I want those bagels in the house. I like them and the children like them and if Tom can't eat them, that's his problem. All he needs to do is use a little strength of character . . . Besides which, I don't think he's that fat. I like him just the way he is."

"Harriet," I said, "I don't think you really want him to lose weight. I think you're frightened of him being thin."

After a pause, Harriet said hesitantly, "Well, sometimes I do think about that and it does scare me . . . Sometimes I think maybe I'll lose him."

Unlikely though it seems, I have heard versions of this story over and over again. It is known about alcoholics that often the spouse doesn't really want the one with the problem to get better. They get something out of the addiction themselves, the dependency or whatever. This is certainly not true in every case, but it is something that merits thought and discussion.

We who have the weight problem must work out our relationships so that the people who care about us know what we need them to do and what we need them to stop doing. Most of the time, if you level with them, tell them you need them to help, they will. It's just that the thin person doesn't really understand the mentality of the fat person. We have to make our weaknesses known. If we can't deal with bagels in the house, then bagels can't come into the house. If a jar of peanut butter takes on the dimensions of a twenty-story peanut-butter skyscraper, then something had better be done about that peanut butter.

What you must realize is that the thin person just doesn't place as much emphasis on food as you do. If you tell him the peanut butter has to go, he probably won't care at all. You are the one who will care, and you have probably been blaming your hesitancy to get the peanut butter out of the house on your mate or on your children, or your parents, or your roommate, or even on the dog.

Let's have a crash course in dealing with this problem. We'll be together every second, and I won't stop talking until you scream for help.

First of all, we have got to enlist the aid and support of your family, whether they're thin or fat. Start out by assuming they want to help you—*even though you think* Billy and Lisa like to have their pizza in the house and Mary is too skinny and needs her food; *even though you think* you can't deprive them of the things they like.

Losing weight is something you've got to do, and you've got to figure out how you can survive doing it and how your family can survive too, without depriving anyone.

First, get rid of the things in the kitchen that will destroy you, the things you cannot cope with. Look in the refrigerator. Probably it is filled with tiny packages of things—leftover tuna-fish salad, baloney, cake, noodles, cheese, cupcakes, chocolate pudding. Let's start here. Let's clean out the refrigerator.

You are someone who should not make your life miserable by having food like that around. You will eat it. Throwing it away will not be wasting food. It will be saving yourself. Besides, there is no place in the refrigerator now to put the food you *can* eat and will-love eating.

Only when you recognize that it is *you* and not your family that is resisting can you move ahead. All of the excuses about Billy and Mary and Lisa are just so much hogwash. It's you putting up roadblocks in front of yourself. The refrigerator is just an extension of you. To attack it, to lay it bare is to make a commitment—to yourself!

Ask your family only what you need to ask of them. Do not punish them with your weight-loss program. No one need be unnecessarily deprived. Get rid of only that food which *you* can't handle. Don't unnecessarily censor what your family eats. On the other hand, tell your spouse or your children or your roommate or your parents how you feel. Let them understand that a mere sentence like "I thought you were on a diet—why are you eating that?"

can cause you enormous harm. What you are doing you have to do on your own, of course, but the input from those around you has got to be positive rather than negative. Certain kinds of "help" are destructive to you. Don't respond with anger. Quietly, calmly, tell the person who said that sentence how it makes you feel: "Please don't say that to me again. For that moment, it makes me hate you, hate myself, and most of all, causes me to eat even more than I had intended. I know it's hard for you to see me doing what you think I shouldn't do, but if you care about me, you'll hold off saying it and we'll both be better off."

If you respond with anger—"Don't say that to me" or "Mind your own business"—they'll never understand what you're trying to do, and you will have created a new conflict. When this happens, the initial problem—helping you to lose weight—is lost in a second argument.

The words "I need your help" are not a sign of weakness but rather of strength. Only the weak never ask for help—they are too afraid to show their need. Try it. Say the words to yourself: I NEED YOUR HELP.

Make it absolutely clear to your family that you don't want to deprive them of anything. They will eat well, and mostly what they want. Be understanding of their needs and try to make them understand yours. If getting your kids a snack in the middle of the afternoon is too difficult for you, tell them. They'll probably be thrilled to make their snack for themselves. (If they do, don't criticize what they've done.)

If your wife brings home donuts for the family and you can't deal with them, tell her. Everyone can live without donuts until you've got your program under control.

If the family is now going to let you off your share of

the kitchen cleaning-up, because that is a hard time for you, then be appreciative of what they are doing. Help more than your share in other areas of the house.

If it kills you that your current girl friend is always cooking up scrumptious fattening things for you, tell her. Maybe she'll take up the challenge and cook you luscious slimming meals.

If you're asking help from friends and family, that means you are bestowing trust upon them. Trust their judgment as well. Listen to what they have to say. Be open-minded. You may reach an impasse—for example, the presence of a jar of peanut butter may be destructive to you, but it may also be your kids' favorite food for lunch. Perhaps a compromise can be found here. Maybe the peanut butter will get hidden where you can't find it. That doesn't sound like too mature a solution, but it can be adequate for the moment. Everyone must be willing to give in—including you. Work together. Plan together. Live together. Have hope together. There's nothing that you can't do when your loved ones are right in there doing it with you.

Chapter VI

How to Deal with Your Friends While You're on the Program

"I think it's just terrific that you've been able to diet like that, but then again you've always had such will power. It's easy for you."

"Oooh, I just think when I look at you, With such a pretty face, how terrific if you could only lose that weight!"

"Well, I'm sure your diet works for you, but frankly, I think you make a mistake not eating between meals. Now, my diet goes like this . . ."

"Oh, come on, forget your diet for a minute. You simply must taste this chocolate cheese cake I've just invented for the club."

"Hey, why are you eating that baked potato? I thought you were on a diet!"

"You're not going on a diet when it's only two weeks till——! (Fill in the blank—Christmas, Passover, the wedding, etc.) Listen, you know you're not going to stay on your diet then, so why pass up the goodies now?"

Well-meaning friends can say the things that give us the greatest pain. But every situation of this type can be handled if you learn to step outside yourself for a moment, turn your immediate anger or irritation under, take a deep breath and say, "Emily, I know you mean well by telling me that I'm looking better today than two months ago, but frankly it hurts my feelings. That time is very clear to me, and I really don't like to be reminded that I looked terrible when I was so fat."

Generally Emily's reaction will be defensive, but it will pass, and you probably won't have to hear anything along those lines again.

The following are suggestions for appropriate responses to this kind of remark:

Remark	*Your Response*
I think it's just terrific that you've been able to diet like that, but then again you've always had such will power. It's easy for you.	Well, it may appear to you that what I've been doing is easy for me. But it isn't. I really don't have any will power. I think our relationship will be much easier if we just don't discuss dieting.
Oooh, I just think when I look at you, With such a pretty face, how terrific if you could only lose that weight!	I know that you have my best interests in mind, but did it ever occur to you that even when I lose all the weight I have to lose I may not have a pretty face? We simply should talk about something other than me and my diet.

Well, I'm sure your diet works for you, but frankly, I think you make a mistake not eating between meals. Now, my diet goes like this . . .

Look, I'm sure your diet is a good one. If it works for you, that's all that's important. Right now, I'm concentrating on my own program, and I don't want to be sidetracked by discussing the pros and cons of our different methods.

Oh, come on, forget your diet for a minute. You simply must taste this chocolate cheese cake I've just invented for the club.

I know you want me to share good things with you, but frankly, it's very hard for me not to eat your cake—and your urging it on me makes it twice as hard. If I want any food when I'm at your home, I promise I'll ask for it. Otherwise, please offer me nothing.

Hey, why are you eating that baked potato? I thought you were on a diet!

I know you care about me but I'm in control of my life and I don't need a policeman. I'll be responsible for my own actions and although I appreciate your concern, it upsets me to have to explain my dieting behavior.

You're not going on a diet when it's only two weeks till _____! (Fill in the blank—Christmas, Passover, the wedding, etc.) Listen, you know you're not going to stay on your diet then, so why pass up the goodies now?

I know that to you food means love and good times and holidays. Well, it means that to me, too, but this year I'm going to have to have a good time without very rich foods. If you love me, you'll help me by encouraging me to stay on my program through this holiday so that next year at this time, I will be able to enjoy the food part too.

The last of the negative attitudes of friends or family is one that doesn't usually require words. It is often seen only in the flicker of an eyebrow, but it says, "So you're doing it again. You know it isn't going to work this time either." No one likes to be defensive, and I know the kind of feelings that rise to the surface when one senses this attitude, but in this case, it is better to leave it all unsaid. Recognize your feelings and know where they come from, then put it all to bed and continue on your way. You're in control, and just because someone thinks that you aren't doesn't make it so.

You will find that your friends will be much more positive and helpful than destructive. Since almost everyone is watching their weight almost all of the time, your friends may go along with you and eat just the way you do when you go out to a restaurant. They will get a kick out of the way you order (see Chapter VIII, Eating Out!) and out of having at least one meal in which calories are controlled. After you've explained the problem your friends will also be supportive when you go to their homes to eat. They will either cook separately for you or make their whole dinner one you can eat, perhaps with some extras for those in the group who are not watching their weight.

Of course, it is really up to you to set the course for your relationship with your friends as it pertains to your eating habits. You cannot keep the fact that you are a food-o-holic a secret, and you cannot keep your program a secret.

We are so used to expecting people to hurt us. We so feel we deserve it because we're fat, because we're weak. We are so accustomed to thinking that our thin friends are somehow better people. We have so many insane negative thoughts about ourselves that we get to the place where we feel we deserve all the bad things said to us and have no right to say, "Whoa, stop, you hurt my feelings."

You have a right to maintain your dignity. You have a right to feel wounded. Look. Listen. No one has a right to demean you, make fun of you, apologize for you, patronize you. It's not your job to look into the intent of your friends when they say things that hurt or embarrass you. Whether or not they think they're doing it for "your good," your only loyalty need be to your own feelings. If they hurt you, tell them—they won't do it again. And maybe when they see that your own dignity is important to you, they'll start viewing you in the same light.

Often when we know someone very well, we take liberties with that person that we wouldn't take with an acquaintance. We sometimes go too far with our "honesty." I'm sure if you looked closely at yourself, you would find that you are as guilty of that as your thin friends are. Truly concerned friends will consider the consequences of their remarks *before* they are spoken, no matter how necessary they think it is for you to hear this "important truth." By their restraint, they will really be helping you and enriching your friendship.

Chapter VII

The Cycle

The cycle is a continuation of the support system. It will help you cope with each food situation, to turn it from trauma into calm. We will learn how to make life easier for ourselves, how to minimize food in our lives and still enjoy it.

Refer back to these sections when you are about to be in any of these food situations until your response becomes automatic.

Planning your meals

Starting at the beginning of the food cycle: plan your meals. We're taking the first step toward not being victimized by our own past life, our own past habits. Remember, we're trying to take the element of chance out of our lives. We're going to try not to leave ourselves vulnerable to anything that can hurt us.

You can plan your meals one day in advance or one week in advance. Try it both ways and see what works out best for you and your schedule. If you're in charge of a family and customarily shop for the week, then meal planning ought to take place before you do your weekly shopping. If you're on the program and your wife is not, sit down with her and plan your meals, incorporating your needs into the list for the whole family. If you live alone, you may prefer once-a-day shopping and perhaps even one-day-in-advance planning. Under no circumstances may you plan your meals any less far ahead than that. Why? It leaves you too vulnerable. You may find yourself suddenly caught without food in the house, and end up rushing to the supermarket and buying all the wrong things because you're shopping while you're starving. You leave the burden of deciding what you're going to put in your mouth for just the wrong time: when you're hungry.

An ideal time to plan the meals for the next day is after you have just finished a good dinner, and you and your family are sitting around the table, feeling comfortable and satisfied with one another. If all the family members are old enough to have a say in food choices, it's a good time for a cooperative atmosphere. Everyone decides together what each would like to eat tomorrow or for the next week in advance. This doesn't mean that everyone is going to eat something different—you're all going to eat similar things, although perhaps slightly different in preparation and definitely in quantity. Breakfast and lunch will certainly be more individual, since most of the time all family members are not eating these meals together.

This is the time to take out your diary. Write in it the foods you will be eating and the calories that you will consume on the following day or through the week. For example, the group may decide that it would like to eat out once or twice this week. Plan accordingly. The group may decide that it wants chicken one night, beef another, a dairy dinner another, fish one night. When this general planning is done, and the shopping list is prepared from the planning, then it is time for you to write very specific quantities and menus into your diary. Those not on the program won't be measuring as you are. There may also be extras they'll be eating that you won't. This way you clearly delineate for yourself what your menu is going to be so that when it is time for the meal, you can check in your diary. You will know what you're going to eat, and you won't have to make last-minute (destructive) decisions . . . "Well, perhaps I'll have a little of this and a little of that."

Planning also means following a basic formula for each meal. For breakfast you want to be sure to include protein (at least one third of your calories), fruit (one third) and some grain (one third).

For lunch, protein should be about two thirds of your calories, the rest in vegetables or fruit.

For dinner, protein should be at least one half of your calories, the rest in vegetables and fruit.

Here are some sample menus that you might write in your diary that illustrate the portions of foods, the calorie counts, and the delicious meals that are possible, even on the 700 calories which this sample includes.

		Calories
Breakfast	1/4 cup of cottage cheese	60
	1/4 cup of sliced peaches	20
	1 ounce of bran cereal	70
		150
Lunch	2 cups of salad greens	20
(home)	1/4 tomato	10
	3 hard-boiled eggs (no yolks)	45
	1 tablespoon of low-calorie Thousand Island dressing	24
	2 tablespoons of cottage cheese	30
	1/4 cup of blueberries	20
		150
Dinner	7 ounces of filet of sole	210
(restaurant)	Salad	10
	Baked potato	100
	Low-calorie Italian dressing	6
	6 stalks of asparagus	30
	10 large strawberries	35
		391
Total for the day		691

Of course, if you are only planning one day in advance, this presumes that you have the necessary foods in the house at least for your first breakfast.

A shopping list for several meals planned in advance might look like this:

Large container of cottage cheese	A dozen eggs
Large cans of cling peaches	Low-calorie dressings
Box of bran cereal	Italian
Various greens for salad (romaine, spinach, Boston, iceberg lettuce, etc.)	Thousand Island
	Blue cheese
	Blueberries
	Chicken breasts
	Chicken legs
	Lean roast
Green peppers	Broccoli
Scallions	Asparagus
Tomatoes	Squash
Onions	Haddock

This list, of course, will cover meals for a number of days, perhaps even for a week. The quantities will depend on how many people are consuming the food. The plan will allow you to handle easily a situation that has probably often been traumatic. We have all found ourselves out of control, rationalizing what we can and cannot eat, what we will and won't eat. How much better to know that all the foods you can eat have been bought and are in your refrigerator. What a relief it is to be sure that your meals are planned, that there are no last-minute decisions to be made. There is no more standing in front of the refrigerator at all hours of the day or night with the frost nipping at your nose, gazing at the myriad possibilities, or going off to a restaurant for lunch or dinner and looking at the menu and wanting everything you know you shouldn't have. There will be no more going to a friend's apartment for dinner and hoping they'll have something low in calories, and finding out that they don't, and ending up eating what they give you. No more stalking around your house, frantically hunting for something to eat.

If you are dining out tonight, you have already planned

your menu, either because you've already been to the restaurant or you've phoned ahead to make sure that *what you want* is available. The phone is a marvelous interceder. There are no printed menus in front of you to send the wrong images into your brain and make you want what you shouldn't have. Instead, you are absolutely focused on what you can eat, and having a marvelously civilized conversation with someone about the availability of what you want in their restaurant. I have found restaurant personnel to be wonderfully cooperative on the phone. As a matter of fact, if your tone and manner are kept warm and help-seeking, you will get practically the attention that a celebrity expects and gets. I do believe that when people find out that you are quite serious about pursuing a healthy life for yourself, they respond with great concern. As a matter of fact, it seems that people will attend you with as much care as you attend yourself. That's an amazing idea because we are inclined to believe that the imposition of our needs on others will produce animosity and make us uncomfortable and embarrassed. Quite the contrary, it produces interest, cooperation and great friendliness. I have established relationships in restaurants with waiters, maître d's, and owners, that would never have come about if I had eaten just what they would ordinarily serve. When you are working things out together, you develop an attitude of mutual interest in the dining process. We all benefit. Friends who take pride in their cooking have responded to my program by producing gourmet meals when I come for dinner. It becomes an exciting treat for me and a real cooking challenge for them.

Planning your meals, preparing your shopping list, knowing where you are going to eat and when . . . all of these things are part of the new pattern of putting yourself in control of your life. This is a sensitive time for you.

You have spent all the years before today building up patterns of behavior and ways of dealing with food that have been destructive to you. Now you're going to start to handle things in a new way. This requires that you develop some really strong support systems to fight against all the old habits that want to jump up and take over your life. Keep up your defense systems:

DON'T
Don't stop planning meals.
Don't shop when hungry.
Don't find yourself without your food in the
house when it's time to eat.
Don't walk into a restaurant without calling first.
Don't visit friends without telling them in advance
of your needs.
Don't put off getting on the scale each morning.
Don't keep it to yourself when someone hurts
your feelings.
Don't leave yourself with large amounts of time
on your hands.
TIME ON YOUR HANDS IS FOOD IN YOUR MOUTH.

Those old habits are waiting. If you let down your defenses, they attack, pushing away the new habits that are just trying to develop a little muscle.

You're going to take control of your life and not be victimized. You're going to know the strong feeling of being free of last-minute decisions when it comes to food, the relief of knowing when you get up in the morning that the food is in the house, the meals are planned. You don't have to worry about it. You've also planned your day. You're a busy person with things to do and people to do them with. Whether you're at home, at work, or at school, all these dangerous pockets of time will be planned. You're going to have elegant healthy meals because that's how you choose to live. And in the process, you're going to lose the weight you desire (whether five pounds or fifty).

As you can see, each step in this program is interwoven with the next. Planning the meals is dependent upon food being in the house, which is dependent on how you make your shopping list, which is dependent on how you structure your day, which is often dependent upon those around you, which is dependent upon the nature of your relationship with friends and family, which is dependent on how well you are able to make your feelings and thoughts known to them, which is dependent upon how you feel about yourself, which is dependent upon how well you did today on your program, which is dependent on how well you planned your meals today.

(1) You will plan your meals AT LEAST ONE DAY IN ADVANCE and, ideally, A FULL WEEK IN ADVANCE.

(2) You will write in your diary exactly what you are going to eat, how many calories it contains, and where you are going to eat it.

(3) You will make up a shopping list for the foods you selected.

(4) You will do your planning with those involved in eating with you.

(5) You will make up your program based on a protein/carbohydrate balance: breakfast, one third protein; lunch, two thirds protein; dinner, one half protein.

(6) You will choose foods that you enjoy eating.

(7) You will go to sleep each night and wake up each morning secure in knowing that you are in control of your life and that a beautiful day awaits you, with myriad pleasures *including eating and losing weight.*

How to shop for food

(1) Never go to the supermarket until your stomach is absolutely prepared: the only time is right after you have eaten! You're calm, reasonable and steady.

(2) Don't enter those dangerous grounds without your very specific, very precise, absolutely enumerated shopping list, the one you made up the night before, after dinner when you were planning your menus for the next day or week.

(3) Go into the supermarket to have a good experience. You are going to be buying foods that are the best-tasting in the store. You are not being deprived! You are carrying out a simple, beautiful plan for good health and delicious eating.

(4) Take your calorie book with brand names with you to the store.

A supermarket is not somewhere to eat. I inevitably see someone pushing his cart and stuffing some fast food into his mouth. That person inevitably is overweight.

My friend Jane is a little person, about five foot one, and since the day she turned twenty-five has been fighting the weight problem. An extra ten pounds for her is a disaster.

One day when she was on one of her usual diets, she and her husband drove to the supermarket. Since they only had to pick up a few things, she told him to wait in the car. Off she went, and of course she got her cart and headed straight for the candy . . . one of those new large Cadbury bars. Ripping the wrapper off, she dug her teeth into the chocolate and then began pushing her cart around the store, trying to concentrate on the shopping and trying to eat the candy bar as fast as she could.

As she turned into one of the aisles, who did she see staring at her with his mouth open? You guessed it. Her husband had decided to come help with the groceries. They stood, momentarily frozen in space. Then Jane finished her bite, pulled herself up to her full five feet one and pushed the cart directly past him, chewing on the candy as though he didn't exist. Neither of them ever mentioned the incident to the other, but the next day she told me that it was the most humiliating moment in her marriage. To be caught redhanded in such a childish caper was almost more than she could bear. The anxiety and potential humiliation just isn't worth it. How many of you have gotten up in the middle of the night and tried to get into the refrigerator without being heard? How many of you have rushed home early to eat something before "they" get home. The truth is, if someone doesn't walk in on you—*you walk in on you!* You are always watching yourself, and because of that I can reason with you and make you see that those secret seconds are really not worth the agony they cause afterward.

Now, for our trip to the supermarket: with stomach and list in order, we enter. Oh, my heavens, what is that odor? I feel my entire body collapsing, my arms and legs being pulled as though I were in a wind tunnel to . . . Aha! It's the bakery counter. Someone must actually be spraying cake odors over our heads to get us. But hold on. They can't do that to us. We're in control here. We just had our good lunch, our filling breakfast—and we're not hungry. We certainly don't eat between meals (where are your commandments?) and if we remember that we're here to win over this store and not to be its victim, we'll pass the bakery counter and not even look. A victory!

On to the vegetables. That's usually first. You can't get into too much trouble here because it's the one place in the supermarket where no one is selling you anything. The vegetables just sit there hoping that someone will recognize that they are probably the most valuable jewels in the shop. This department can really make your diet. These are low-calorie items, they're delicious, they're beautifully formed and they're many-colored. Each of those characteristics in its turn performs a wonderful function at the table.

Vegetables cost least when they are in season, and that's when they are the most delicious. A good way to vary your menu is to focus on the vegetables in season— save some money and have a more tasty treat. A large platter of summer tomatoes, sliced and doused with pepper, dill and chives is superb. As I write this, broccoli has never been cheaper or better, as is true of summer squash.

Let's move on to the dairy counter. Take a dozen eggs home with you, a carton of skimmed milk. By the way, take notice of the label here. Does it say skimmed milk or does it say low-fat milk? Many of us have been deceived into thinking they're one and the same. They're not! Skimmed milk has 80 calories a cup; low-fat milk, 110 calories to 160 calories a cup.

Nothing makes our life easier than when calories are marked on containers. Soon all food products will be marked in that manner. Look for cottage cheese, for example that contains 50 to 60 calories per quarter cup, or 100 to 120 calories per half cup. That's just right for our program.

To the poultry counter. Buy chicken breasts and legs, or, when available, turkey legs. Always watch for the special and when they come, buy a lot, take them home cook them and freeze in individual portions. A breast that weighs about 5½ ounces has about 1/2 ounce of bone, so it's about 250 calories (at 50 calories an ounce). That's just about right for chicken as an entree. If you want to make sure that you know exactly what you have eaten, weigh the piece before you eat. Then weigh the bones after you've eaten and you'll know many ounces you've consumed. I must confess, I still do this every time I have chicken.

When you pass the condiment area, pick up some onion powder, which is a good basic seasoning for the dieter, and some dill, which is wonderful in salads, and other herbs that please you.

At the canned goods counter, buy several cans of tuna fish packed in water (100 calories for three ounces). Keep some in your office, and when you eat lunch at your desk, order some garden salad and onion. Combine these with the tuna and you have a gourmet luncheon.

At the canned fruit section, pick up the very large cans of sliced cling peaches or fruit cocktail. (We'll explain how to prepare them on page 78.) Here's where we fool them. You see they keep all the larger cans at the bottom of the counter; they are generally cheaper. They think we don't want to bend down and that we'll therefore buy the most expensive size. Wrong. Not only will we bend down, but we will do a separate bend for each can. It's cheaper, and it's terrific for our waistline.

Now, to the frozen foods section. Vegetables galore at all times of the year. Be careful of the ones in sauces. Check the calories. Perhaps it's something you could schedule for a later meal. Some supermarkets have large bags of plain vegetables—broccoli, green beans, Brussels sprouts, cauliflower. This is a wonderful, relatively inexpensive way to keep vegetables on hand.

Also at the frozen foods counter, check the frozen fish

fillets. Shrimp, mackerel, sole, haddock and flounder are all low in calories (about 20 calories to an ounce, raw; 30 calories per ounce when broiled or baked).

The cereal counter is an important stop. Look for the cereals that are high in fiber—the brans—low in calories (60 or 70 per ounce) and high in nutrition. Read those labels. It is an education. The consumer is finally beginning to benefit from the labeling process. By the way, a new product has emerged—bread that advertises an enormous amount of fiber at just 50 calories an ounce. This is absolutely something you could work into your program with some satisfaction. The fiber is in the form of cellulose, and when you eat it along with some liquid, you get quite a full feeling.

Check your list. Keep a pencil in your hand all through the market. Get everything on the list, nothing that isn't there. Now onward to the check-out counter.

This is a terrific time for you. Look into everyone's carts to see what they contain. Try to figure out what the owner looks like from the contents. Let's see . . . this one has steaks, bagels, preserves, crackers, tomatoes, pretzels, diet soda, magazines, cheeses . . . Uh huh. Could take off about twenty-five, right? This one's got yogurt, veal, strawberries, potatoes, vegetables and whole-wheat bread—he's looking pretty healthy and thin. And this one: cottage cheese, tuna, peaches, chicken, broccoli, squash, tomatoes, radishes—why, he must be the healthiest, happiest person I've ever seen. It's you, of course. We made it. Our list checks out. We're not hungry, the bill is a lot less than what it used to be, and we're feeling a little superior to those around us. It's okay. Feel superior—you deserve it. You just added another victory to your list.

Let's take the time here to talk about those of you who are put in the position of buying foods that you cannot eat, a subject partially covered in the chapter "How to Deal with Your Family."

The question here is: what foods can you handle? If you can stand to have cake or peanut butter or the bread your family wants in the house but can't get too close to them, then when it's time to shop for such food, let them buy it themselves. *You* can't buy it.

Preparing food for eating and storage

If you are the one who is on the program and in charge of the food, for yourself or for a family, there is no doubt that the less time you spend in the kitchen and the less time you spend with food altogether, the better off you are.

Now you have just returned from the supermarket with all the food, and are ready to put it away. This is the time to kill two birds with one you-know-what. Prepare what foods you can before you put them away, and get all this over with.

The important points here are:

(1) Buy in large quantities. Your house should be run as much like a restaurant as possible.

(2) Cook in large quantities. Cook up the chicken, for example, all in one enormous batch. It saves a lot of time in the kitchen. It takes no longer to prepare eight chicken breasts and four turkey drumsticks than it does one or two.

(3) Freeze in large quantities. Take your chicken out of the oven, instantly wrap each piece in its own aluminum foil and pop it into the freezer, leaving out just what you're going to have for tonight's dinner. If you freeze

chicken while it's hot, when you defrost, it is still moist and tender. It's a good idea to label the packages for contents and weight before they're frozen. This helps you choose the proper amount when you're defrosting for dinner.

(4) Prepare ongoing things like salad in large quantities. Get all the cleaning, chopping and paring over at one time. Keep your salad in large Baggies or medium-size garbage bags, or use attractive clear plastic bowls. The clear concept is so you can readily see when you need to begin refilling. Keep plastic containers and bags on hand for storage.

Why all this mass preparation? For one thing, so that when it is time to eat a meal, no elaborate preparations are necessary. Just defrost the chicken or stick a 2-cup measure into the salad bag, and *voilà!* you have a wonderful main course or a smashing salad. The longest anything should take you is a few minutes to steam some fresh vegetables which have been cleaned and prepared before going into the refrigerator. In no time a terrific meal is in front of you, in fact, in less time than it would have taken you to order it in a restaurant and be served.

Of course, there is more to all this than just the instant-ready concept. It is that with extra food around, temptation is indeed again at the door. It doesn't take much to rationalize and say, "Another piece of chicken can't hurt. After all, it's protein—not like cake or ice cream."

Well, another piece of chicken can be 250 calories, more than half your dinner allotment. Besides, we're trying to train ourselves to eat only when we sit down at the table, to put everything we're going to eat on our plate and eat only that. Eating the extra piece of chicken means we have either munched on it standing up at the kitchen counter or that we have entered the kitchen after we have served the meal and taken something additional to our plate.

Let's talk now about cooking. The idea is to allow the true flavor of the food to make direct contact with your taste buds, without fancy—and fattening—sauces, dressings, butters and creams. You will notice that we don't cook with salt, either. Recent findings indicate that Americans use far more salt than their bodies need. In this program, we don't season with salt at all, but rely on the salt that is naturally in the food itself.

For example, fish is one of the more glorious foods in the world. There is no need for butter or oil to make fish delicious. Take your striped bass, or bluefish, or sole or turbot, sprinkle with some onion powder, paprika and pepper, and place under the broiler. With thin fillets, your fish is done in about five to seven minutes. For a thick, juicy striped bass, broil for five minutes and then turn over for another three or four. Don't overcook fish. It spoils the flavor and the texture. Another extremely simple preparation calls for cutting up carrots, celery, onions, green peppers, putting them into a large pan, covering with water and laying either your fillet or a whole fish on top. Cover for fifteen minutes and poach. The fish takes on the lovely, delicate flavor of the vegetables, and they make a good low-calorie accompaniment to the dish.

As to chicken, I prepare it in large quantities. Buy eight chicken breasts. Skin them. That's right, remove the skin and as much of the fat as possible. Then cut the breasts in half and wash them well in cold water.

Line a large, shallow baking pan with foil and place the chicken breasts, flesh side up, in the pan. Sprinkle with lots of paprika, onion powder and pepper. Slide under the broiler (not you, the chicken) for five minutes.

Set the timer, for heaven's sake—that's another invention that's been provided to make life easier. At the end of five minutes, turn the chicken, add more paprika, onion powder and pepper. Put back under the broiler for five minutes.

At the end of five minutes, put the pan into the oven and bake for forty minutes at 350°. Your chicken will be beautifully golden-brown, the breast side will be russet-colored and crisp because it's been cooking face down throughout the process. Best of all, when you eat the chicken (which is not now) you will find it to be as moist and delicious as though it had been cooked with the skin on.

Now, while it is still hot, wrap each individual piece in aluminum foil and put into your freezer. Only keep as much chicken in the refrigerator as you're going to use tonight.

While the chicken has been cooling, you have been preparing your salad bags or bowls. In one bowl or bag, you will be placing the "innards" of the salad: sliced zucchini, radishes, red cabbage, green peppers, red peppers, celery. I don't include cucumber in the advance preparation because it does not keep well; it becomes transparent and then soggy. If you like cucumber, slice some into your salad just before serving. In the second bowl or bag, place the leafy part of the salad—Boston leaf or iceberg lettuce, endive, spinach. Wash it carefully, tear into bite-size pieces, drain and place in the bag or bowl. Make very large amounts that will last at least four or five days for lunch and/or dinner. It's marvelous, because when it's time to eat, and you're hungry, you just take your 2-cup measuring cup, dip it into the crunchy bowl and then into the leafy vegetables, and there's your salad. Garnish it with some sliced tomato, cucumbers or onion.

For protein in your salad, you might like to add hard-boiled eggs. Boil the eggs right before it's time to eat, if you like them hot. Or cook up a dozen eggs when you are doing your initial salad preparation, and then they're ready too. *Remember, we just eat the egg whites and discard the yolks.* Egg whites, 15 calories; egg yolks, 60. One whole egg, 75 calories.

As to vegetable preparation, if you bought a whole cauliflower, clean it, separate the flowerets and store in a large bowl or bag in the refrigerator.

My favorite cauliflower dish: slice the flowerets, along with some red and green peppers and onions. Heat a wok and toss in the vegetables at very high heat. Then add a little chicken bouillon and soy sauce. This is an offshoot of the Chinese stir-fry method, and the result is a colorful and delicious low-calorie dish—30 calories to the cup.

As to broccoli, let's talk for a moment about broccoli al dente. First, it contains only 30 calories a stalk and it can be cooked simply by tossing over a little heat in the wok. Watch that it doesn't burn. It can be eaten raw in a salad or barely steamed with a little lemon and pepper. By the way, exactly the same recipe can be used for cauliflower.

Summer squash is another calorie bargain at 30 calories a cup. Cut it in chunky slices with some sweet white onion, and cook for ten or fifteen minutes in a pot large enough to handle quite a lot at one time. Freeze the extra portions for later meals. When you serve it, add a little pepper or cinnamon.

I believe that most vegetables should be cooked so as to stay as close to what nature gives us in the garden as possible. Don't peel vegetables. The fiber is in the skin, and the more fiber you take into your system, the better your insides will work. The exception would be that the waxy surface on some cucumbers is probably not good for you.

Raw zucchini makes a wonderful addition to a salad. If you're splurging on winter squash, mash it and add a little vanilla and cinnamon for a lovely flavor.

For asparagus, cut off the white ends and trim off any brown crusts. Trim the ends of scallions if they are bruised. Radishes: clean and store whole. Green beans: snap off the long string at one end; wash and store. The principle is the same: clean the vegetables as soon as you get home and store in plastic bags or containers. By the way, all these vegetables except for the asparagus are delicious raw as well. If you've never tried them, try them.

About fruit . . . Don't wash fresh fruit before you put it away; it keeps better dry. If you want to keep a container of canned sliced peaches or peach halves or fruit cocktail in the refrigerator, this is a good time to open a large can of fruit, drain off the syrup, place the fruit in a colander and wash it. And wash it and wash it. Put it in a container and add some cold water, and it's ready to eat. (Every time you use the fruit, pour off the water and put some fresh water in. That keeps the amount of syrup in the water down and the calories down in turn.

Keep a pad and pencil somewhere convenient in the kitchen so that as you use up something like the paprika or the last of the green peppers, you can easily mark it down, and when it's time for the next shopping spree your list is practically prepared.

The marvelous thing about what we're doing is that we're caring a great deal about what we are feeding ourselves, about how it looks and tastes, but that it is taking very little of our time. We are making certain that when we look into our refrigerator, it is not a sad sack of an icebox, containing only the remnants of a squashed tomato or a clammy puckered cucumber, showing us that the punishment is in force: we need to lose weight, so we're in prison and are being treated like prisoners. On the contrary, food is very much a part of our life, but it's in the proper perspective. Everyone likes to eat, you and I are no exception. But we are learning to eat as well as everyone else and still be kind to ourselves. You will find out that you are eating healthier and better than your friends. In fact, it will be they who will want all your recipes, who will start duplicating the way you are shopping, preparing food and eating—the way you are living. There is no deprivation here, only exhilaration.

Serving food

Whether you live alone, are the mother of a family or a husband who generally leaves such matters to his wife— what a lovely time this can be. The culmination of calorie planning, of expert cooking, of concern for proper nutritional balance, of concern for appearance. Now the artist in you (and the mathematician too) goes to work.

Here's a sample dinner menu:

6 ounces of chicken	300
1 cup of salad	10
1 tablespoon of Italian low-calorie dressing	6
1 cup of summer squash	30
2 tablespoons of cottage cheese	25
1/4 cup of peaches	20
total	391

(1) You have weighed and marked the chicken breast after you cooked it. You know it is 6 1/2 ounces. Figuring about a half ounce for the bone, you have 6 ounces of lovely chicken breast.

(2) Take a cup measure and dip it into the salad you have already prepared. Add the dressing. The way the food looks on the plate should not disappoint you. So plan your meals for color and texture: the crisp, chewy, texture and varied colors of the salad contrast beautifully with the yellow squash and the crusty russet glow of the chicken.

(3) Dip your cup measure into the steamed squash (page 77), making sure you pour off the liquid so that you are really getting a full cup, You will be amazed at just how much squash one cup contains and at how filling it is.

(4) Take a dessert plate and measure out 2 tablespoons of cottage cheese and 1/4 cup of washed and drained sliced peaches. Add some vanilla and sweetener to the cottage cheese. Place the peaches on top and sprinkle with some cinnamon.

(5) Prepare a tall frosty glass of water with ice cubes glistening in it and put it at your place at the table.

(6) Place your plate on the table and take your seat.

(7) Now look at what you have done: prepared an absolutely beautiful meal and served it to someone special, namely you. No one deserves it more!

If you are in the position of serving others than yourself —family, friends—remember that the amounts they want and need and the way they like their food flavored *can vary enormously.*

There are two ways this can be handled. You yourself can decide how much they get—how many pieces of chicken, who gets butter on their vegetable. Or serve buffet style, either from the dining room or the kitchen. This way, you take your own portioned meal on your plate and let the others serve themselves however they like. You don't have to be exposed to the addition of butter to vegetables or sour cream to potatoes or whatever the others choose to do with their basic meal. Your family or guests should never feel that you are imposing a "diet" on them. Rather, you are preparing lovely meals that offer them a choice.

As I mentioned earlier, if your family wants things that you cannot handle, then let them know that the food is on the buffet table, but that they have to get it themselves. If you can't deal with watching them eat it, then you had better get that out now too so that comfortable eating arrangements can be handled. For example, you might leave the dining-room table before dessert.

However you choose to serve the meal, you will be pleased by the exclamations at the sight of the beautifully, carefully conceived dinner. Any stranger walking into your home at this moment would never guess that someone in the family is being extremely cautious about what he is eating, in this instance, a 400-calorie dinner.

The real lesson in self-control for those of you who have done the cooking and serving is to learn to banish the following sentences from your vocabulary:

"Isn't this chicken delicious, dear? Do you want some more?" "Can I get you some more salad?" "Would you like a second helping of squash?" "Does anyone want any more of anything?"

You no longer offer anything but the initial platter of food or the attractive buffet, which is out for anyone to see. If someone wants something more, he can get up and get it—if there is more. You will not subject yourself to the pain of having to serve more food that you cannot have. Whether the people around the table are children or grownups, they are all capable of going to the kitchen or to the buffet table for seconds, if they desire them. It's their responsibility. Your responsibility ended when you served this nutritious, delicious meal.

Of course, this information must be out in the open; it can't be a secret feeling that you have. Tell everyone the new rule—let them share your needs. Explain why it is so hard for you to give them seconds. Reassure them that there is enough food for them, that you have considered them in the preparation. You have probably even prepared foods for the buffet table that you can't eat at all —a potato dish or rice.

Now, let's sum up the serving of the meal:

(1) Open your diary to the proper page and place it somewhere convenient in the kitchen to note what portions you have allowed yourself for this meal.

(2) Measure and portion out the food, giving yourself exact amounts as indicated, and if you are serving others, giving them portions appropriate to their needs and desires. Arrange the food on the plates so that it's pleasing in color and texture. Or

(3) Set up a buffet table in the kitchen or dining room so that the others can serve themselves.

(4) Do not offer second helpings to anyone; let them serve themselves.

(5) Make certain you have explained all your rules to friends and family.

(6) Notice that you are not deprived. You have a beautiful plate of food in front of you that you are entitled to, that you have planned and prepared. You are exhibiting gorgeous control of your food and your life.

(7) Notice that no one else is deprived at your table. Friends and family will have delicious meals and all they choose to eat.

Eating the meal

What a victory! Being able to sit down and eat a delicious meal without feeling guilty or conspicuous.

No more "tiny tastings of this and that" or "I'm not really hungry, buts." No more leaving a table hungry because you're not on a diet but you're too embarrassed to eat what you need to stop those terrible gnawing pains that you have always interpreted as meaning that you were still starving. Now you're a person who sits down to a meal that is beautifully prepared, delicious and healthy, that is in your calorie range, that looks like a thin person's dinner. What a lovely way to set the tone for the meals. You don't have to concern yourself with anything other than enjoying the results of your precise planning.

Take your seat at the table. This is the place you have designated as *your* eating place in your house. This place and no other. No more eating in bed, on the living-room sofa or standing in the kitchen. Just here in your comfortable chair at the table. The place that is yours and no one else's. That's a nice feeling, too.

Take a good look at the food on the plates and the others at your table. Take a deep breath and feel how wonderful it is to have such good friends and family and the access to such good food. You might try putting your elbows on the table, clasping your hands together and leaning your chin on them as you watch the pleasure of everyone's face as they eat the tempting meal you have produced again today.

Wait till everyone else has begun to eat, and then take a couple of sips of your water or iced tea, holding the glass in both hands in a relaxed position. Take note of this position, as you are going to assume it a number of times during the meal. We'll call it the "time-out" position.

Now replace your glass and take your fork and spear something with it, a piece of squash, a crunch of salad. Taste it, know it. No shoveling. Easily, calmly let it enter your mouth, chew it so that you know you have indeed just eaten something and that the sensation was clear and true. Notice your posture and everyone else's. Notice how certain people surround their food with their bodies; they bend over it, even take their arm with the utensil in it and surround their plate, then curl their eating implement around to them almost in the position of being fed by someone else. I'm convinced that this posture comes from earliest times, when man guarded his food so that no one would take it from him. However, it wouldn't surprise me if this same position is used in hopes that others can't really see the plates from which we shovel in the food. To make the eating experience pleasant for everyone, you'll want to be bringing the food to you instead of taking your mouth to the food!

If you can, cross your legs in a casual manner, as you might if you were having a conversation. What this position will do is place you even further back from the table and help you stay relaxed. It almost makes you feel as though you don't care whether you eat or not. You will notice that thin people assume this posture at the dinner table, and probably it does indicate their attitude toward their food—one that we would do well to simulate.

Take a few bites. Taste the chicken and put down your fork. Use this time to savor the food, taste it and chew it again. Push your back into your chair and take another relaxing deep breath. Continue in this manner, with your breathing times, eating times, times-out. Establish a fixed but restful and calming pattern to your meal.

(1) Time-out
(2) Eating
(3) Concentrated breathing
(4) Eating
(5) Time-out
(6) Eating
(7) Concentrated breathing
(8) Eating . . . etc.

You'll find you're enjoying your meal much more and taking longer to eat than almost anyone at the table. Your stomach has time to signal you that it is getting the food, and by the end of the meal you will really understand that you have eaten well and eaten enough. Finally, you will be feeling extremely satisfied with yourself because you have again exhibited such gorgeous control over your life.

What a nice thought also when you finish your meal to know that you will be able to eat at least this well forever. Imagine, if you're getting all this satisfaction from as little as 700 to 1000 calories a day, what next?

By the way, for the times when you're out and others may order drinks or appetizers before the meal and you have not included an appetizer for yourself for this meal, order an iced tea, club soda or hot tea—anything that you can sit and "play with" so that you keep yourself occupied. Ask for lemon for the tea, perhaps sweetener. With the club soda, perhaps get some lime or lemon. Busy yourself with the preparation, and then drink it slowly. You'll find this also eases any hunger pangs or anxiety pangs you may be having. The time should pass easily, but if your dinner partners are intent on waiting too long a time before a meal, then tell them that you would like to order. You'll find that they will usually want to join you. They've probably just been carried away by your scintillating conversation and haven't realized that it's time to eat. Again, state your need, softly and gently, and it will be heard and dealt with in the same way.

At the close of the meal drink coffee or tea. Sipping is a fabulous way to sit out the times when dinner partners might want to linger over after-dinner liqueurs or desserts. Tea seems to signal that the meal has come to an end, as other foods or an excruciatingly full feeling used to—in your former life!

Cleaning up after the meal

I wish this chapter didn't have to exist at all. This is such a dangerous time. If you don't have to be the one to do this chore, then terrific. You don't even have to read the rest of this chapter.

If there is food left over from the meal, it must immediately be packaged and refrigerated or frozen. Opaque plastic containers with tight-fitting lids are just the thing for this process. Food is neither easily seen nor easily removed from the refrigerator when it is packed away. You should have plastic containers in all sizes for freezing and storing.

While you are putting things away, don't allow yourself even one taste of anything. Remember, you have finished eating. You only eat sitting down at the table. You do not ever eat standing up in the kitchen. Eating time is over. We are trying to develop new patterns of behavior. We do not now eat between meals, and this period after the meal is over is indeed "between meals."

I think you might find it helpful to put on rubber gloves for the cleaning-up process. They come in comfortable styles and sizes now for men and women. They protect your hands and nails from the soap and water, and they also discourage you from falling into the old habits of picking up food at this particularly sensitive time.

After all extra food is put away, scrape the plates quickly into the trash bag or into the disposal. Think of the leftovers on the plates as garbage. They are not edible. As a matter of fact, if you have to convince youself that everyone you know has a communicable disease—do so. Pretend that if you even touch their food with your fingers, you will come down with a severe malady. (And if you're really kind to your dogs and cats, you won't poison them either with table scraps and leftovers. They too have had their rations and will eat as you will—at their next meal.)

Now that all food has either been thrown away or stored, the kitchen and dining room are safe. It's a matter of you or your dishwasher going to work to do the rest. BUT DO IT NOW! Get it done. Clean the kitchen and know that when you walk out of there, you don't have to go back in again until preparation for the next meal. Don't put it off. If you sit down with company after dinner, and they stay until eleven or even two in the morning, and then you have to go into the kitchen to clean up—you will rekindle again all the old eating feelings. It is disastrous to put off the cleaning process.

Explain this to the people you've eaten with. Somebody will almost certainly volunteer to help you. Men who are entertaining still seem to get such offers of help more than women. Whatever your sex, say yes. It can make the cleaning-up process less tedious; it will pass quickly and you'll still be part of the evening.

Let's restate these steps:

(1) Clean the kitchen *immediately* after you get up from the dining table.
(2) Make sure all extra foods are put into containers and stored.
(3) Put on rubber gloves.
(4) Scrape plates.
(5) Understand that those leftovers are poison.

You've gotten through the whole cycle and won. The world is your oyster. All things are possible for you, beginning with being thin and being in control of your life.

Chapter VIII

Eating Out

Coffee shops, diners and fast-food places

The experience of even being in this kind of eatery will be the hardest for you. These are the places you always used to like to go to before you were being kind to yourself. "Fast foods" mean lots of carbohydrates, everything fried with fat, potatoes included at no charge, and fat, fat, fat. All the wrong things are displayed under glass and, to make it worse, there isn't the flexibility of ordering that there would be in a larger restaurant.

You can control the situation and even enjoy it by following the program.

Don't pick up a menu! Before you walk in, check your diary and see what you have written for today. Did you anticipate being in this coffee shop? Then you did plan your meal. What have you written? It's lunchtime and you planned a tossed salad and tuna fish.

Okay, a tossed salad. Almost certainly any place will have a tossed salad except a hamburger joint, etc. (Hamburgers, etc., are not for you at this time of your life. The tiniest hamburger served in a fast-food emporium is 250 calories. The milk shakes are 250 calories, and so are the small French fries.) You can't eat in those places. Just pretend during this time in your life that they don't exist, and don't go near them. If someone you're with wants to go in, let him go. Don't even walk in. It's too hard on you and you shouldn't have to deal with it.

As to coffee shops, in most towns they will have individual cans of tuna. However, when they do, the tuna is usually packed in oil.

Even though we don't like to do this, let's substitute. As a matter of fact, when you're planning ahead it's a good idea to take a special page in your diary and write down what you might eat should you end up in a coffee shop for breakfast, lunch or dinner. Then when you're in the unexpected situation, you can just turn to that page, and this menu also is already planned.

For example, these are things the fast-food shops generally have on hand that you can use to plan meals in advance:

	Food	*Calories*
BREAKFAST	Dry cereals in individual boxes	70
	Skimmed milk (4 ounces)	40
	Whole milk (4 ounces)	75
	Banana	90
	Egg	75
	Cottage cheese (2 tablespoons)	25
LUNCH	Hard-boiled egg (just the white)	15
	Cottage cheese (2 tablespoons)	25
	Tossed salad (no dressing)	10

	Tomato (2 slices)	15
	Onion	5
	Banana	90
	Canteloupe	50
	Apple	70
DINNER	(This is a hard one because generally everything is fried or breaded or in gravies or sauces—but you can do it.)	
	Chicken (2 slices)	200
	Turkey (2 slices)	200
	Tuna (drained, about 3 1/2 ounces)	150
	Tossed salad (no dressing)	10
	Lettuce	10
	Tomato (2 slices)	15
	Onion	5
	Cottage cheese (2 tablespoons)	25
	Fresh fruit	65–70

For lunch, you might combine cottage cheese, egg whites, the tossed salad, tomatoes and onion for a delicious salad. For dinner you might combine the turkey or chicken and the fresh vegetables to create a chef's salad.

Don't use the house dressing, please. Make your own with vinegar, pepper and onion. If they have onion or garlic powder, your salad dressing can turn into something quite tasty.

Write all of these possibilities in your diary, and then you'll know that wherever you are, no matter what roadside coffee shop or big-city coffee shop or little-town coffee shop, you can get a decent meal for yourself, one you'll be happy eating. And when you've finished, you'll feel satisfied. You've handled this extremely difficult situation ... and succeeded again. Walk out of that coffee shop and know you're a winner!

A good restaurant

The scenario of my own early experience on the program at a fine restaurant may be instructive.

At The Press Box

The waiter approaches the table and asks my friend and me if we want drinks. She is not on the program but says no anyway and I, of course, say the same. Do we want to order now? Yes, indeed.

ME: I would like you to have the chef prepare a platter that consists of the following things . . .

WAITER: (Looks at me, smiling, hand poised on his pad)

ME: . . . six shrimp, two whole, unsliced hard-boiled eggs . . .

WAITER: (Still not writing, but his expression has changed from smiling to confusion and annoyance)

ME: Three slices of tomato, some slices of—

WAITER: (Still hasn't written) You want what?

ME: I would like six shrimp, two hard-boiled eggs, but please don't have them sliced. I would like them whole. About three slices of tomato, some slices of onion.

WAITER: Raw onion? (Starts writing—still a little confused, but getting into it)

ME: Yes. Some capers if you have them. Cucumbers if you have any around. And one of your small bowls of mixed salad.

WAITER: (Getting a little hysterical) Salad. You want a salad.

ME: Yes, you see, what we want to do is have these

WAITER: lovely ingredients you're going to bring us and we want to cut them up, add some salad and toss it all together. We're counting calories and this is all we can have—no more, no less.

WAITER: (Smiling) Oh, yes, oh, yes. I see.

ME: Now for the dressing, we have a problem because we can't have any oil. But I thought if you have some garlic . . .

WAITER: And some lemon.

ME: Yes, lemon if you think that's good, some vinegar, pepper. We just can't have salt or oil.

WAITER: Leave it to me. (Eyes twinkling) I have an idea. We'll come up with something.

He leaves. My friend picks up the menu which we have not yet looked at. I tell her I never look at a menu until after I've ordered (because, as you must know, I planned this meal before I even entered this restaurant). We look and she asks about various appetizers, and I say why I wouldn't order them, primarily because I couldn't be exactly certain of the calories, and I'm not taking chances. I will not put myself into the hands of strangers and trust them, when their primary concern is not *my* health.

My friend points to a spinach salad with bacon, mushrooms and scallions and asks, Couldn't we have that? Yes, I say, but the bacon is absolutely not allowable. We could have our waiter give us the raw spinach instead of the salad greens for our salad, and we could have the raw mushrooms and scallions, too. She instantly gets the waiter's attention and tells him we would like to have one spinach salad with mushrooms and scallions, no bacon or dressing, and that we will divide that as our greens. He understands perfectly and leaves our table with great enthusiasm and purpose. In a short time he returns with the most gorgeous platter of shrimp, two whole hard-boiled eggs, three slices of tomato, all beautifully arranged, with dark-green capers in the center. He places between us a large spinach salad and brings us two wooden bowls.

ME: Cut up everything into small pieces, as you would to make a salad at home. Don't forget to remove the yolks from the eggs.

MY FRIEND: Remove the yolks? I can't do that. I can't eat just the whites of the egg. And I don't want to cut up the salad. Why can't I just eat it right off the platter?

ME: You can. Go ahead. Eat the yolks. I don't eat yolks. An egg is 75 calories. The yolk is 60 and is filled with cholesterol. The whites are 15 calories and contain the protein. I love to have egg whites in a salad and I want to make a tossed salad. You are free to do what you want.

MY FRIEND: No . . . I want to do it exactly like you're doing it. I want to at least try it.

How vehemently people protest when you suggest that they approach familiar foods in a new way. The hard-boiled-egg syndrome is constant. "How can you throw away the yolks? Eggs are too expensive. I can't eat the whites without the yolks. Uggghhh." Grownup actually walk around saying "Uggghhh" when you mention fish or cottage cheese or eggs without yolks! Their approach to food is very much like a child's—as a matter of fact, the fat person is probably still eating like a child or still fantasizing about certain foods the same way as when he was a child. For example, how do you feel about a grownup eating a Hostess Twinkie? Picture yourself eating one of those or one of whatever it is that you eat. Now picture me looking at you eating your Hostess Twinkie? Feel comfortable? I hope not.

To get back to the restaurant, and to summarize the action: by the time we finish preparing our salad our waiter returns to the table with a self-satisfied Charlie Chaplin, "I'm on top of this situation" look. He brings with him a tray of ingredients and prepares a salad dressing of his own invention.

ME: How many cloves of garlic?

WAITER: Three.

He takes our individual salads, adds garlic, fresh lemon juice, wine vinegar and pepper and tosses with great abandon. When he's served each of us, he steps back.

He waits. We taste.

ME: It's wonderful—it's that garlic. Did you press it yourself?

WAITER: Yes.

MY FRIEND: I love it. (She is now lost in wonder at her 150-calorie salad, without oil, without egg yolks and without salt)

The waiter stands gazing at us in silence, as though he had created not just the dressing, not just the salad, but us as well. We and our satisfied happiness are his total creation. We have absolutely made his day, I am sure. Before we leave, he returns to the table and says, "You come back and I will do that for you again, exactly."

I have had similar experiences in a dozen different restaurants in a dozen different cities. If you send out positive feelings to the waiter—gentle voice, gentle manner, but firm and unswerving—the response will be better than you can imagine.

Approach the restaurant with the view that they are going to supply you with what you can eat, but that you are going to accomplish this in a cooperative manner. You need the waiter's help, and you will get it if you know what you are doing, if you explain your problem clearly and if you stay calm. When you get what you asked for, make sure you act appreciative and thank the waiter. The next time you go to that restaurant will be easier and even more fun. The waiter really does want to please you, and if he thinks he's also being creative and inventive, his ego is having a good time too.

Eating out is a terrific time, providing you've checked the restaurant in advance and know what you can get so that you don't feel deprived. In fact, you will feel special. A good formula for eating dinner out is to order:

Fish, no butter
Baked potato, no butter
Salad with a dressing like the one the waiter made in the preceding scenario
A green vegetable, without butter
Fresh strawberries or melon, or another fresh fruit in season

That is a superb meal. Now that you are on the program you will learn to love to eat fish. Be brave enough to try as many different kinds as possible, and—make sure they are cooked without oil or butter.

Bear in mind that it is easier to stay on the program in a Chinese restaurant than in almost any other ethnic restaurant. Get hold of the menu ahead of time, if possible, or phone to make sure they have chicken, shrimp or beef with vegetables, a really low-calorie dish. Ask them to leave out the cornstarch in the cooking. Steamed fish are also delicious and low in calories and side dishes of vegetables like broccoli are marvelous when cooked Chinese style. Just make certain, again, that all dishes are without cornstarch. Side dishes of bean sprouts or chicken, shrimp, beef or vegetables with bean sprouts are all low-calorie.

Go out to dinner, but remember:

(1) Check the restaurant ahead of time.

(2) Know what you're going to order in advance.

(3) Order without looking at the menu.

(4) Stay calm and easy when giving your order so that you can get the waiter's cooperation.

(5) Stay ever vigilant: no butter, please: please broil it dry: no oil, please.

(6) Enjoy. You are not a deprived person. You are a special person having an exceptionally special dinner.

Eating out at a friend's house

If you're invited to a friend's house for dinner, before you accept you must ask what is on the menu. If they are serving something you can't eat, ask if they would mind if you ate at home and came over after dinner. Or else you might ask if they would mind if you brought your own dinner. Either of these will work out fine, but usually the host or hostess will say, "Well, I'm having Chicken Cacciatore, but I can keep a piece of chicken out for you without the sauce. And instead of putting hollandaise sauce on the asparagus, I can serve yours plain, and the salad too. And can you have fresh fruit for dessert?"

Your friends enjoy making you comfortable. It isn't that hard for them and, after all, the real basis of getting together is not the food but your friendship. Remember, however, it's not up to them to be responsible for you and your program, it's up to you. Though they may have the best intentions, they may not feed you exactly the right things. It's your job to watch that and to keep them from feeling they have harmed you.

A friend on the program described to me a weekend he spent with friends in Connecticut. Before Dave left, he phoned his hostess and described exactly what he could eat. "Fine," the hostess said, and off Dave went for the weekend.

He sat with her in the kitchen Saturday afternoon and asked what she was preparing for dinner. "Lobster Savannah," she said. "You're going to love it." "Lobster Savannah?" he gasped. "Isn't that the recipe where the meat is taken out of the lobster and stuffed back in with cream and all sorts of wonderful things?" Noticing the strange expression on his face, she asked, "You can eat that, can't you?"

Well, he persuaded her to leave his lobster plain, untouched, unstuffed, un-Savannahed.

At dinner each of the guests had Lobster Savannah, and Dave had his plain boiled lobster. Twenty minutes later the others had finished their fifty-million-calorie meal, and Dave was only halfway through his lobster. They sat and talked, and still he ate. They had some coffee, and more lobster remained before him. By that time, the entire table was aware that the hundred-calorie lobster had taken three times longer to eat than the fifty-million-calorie job. Whether he's right or not, Dave believes he enjoyed his more than they enjoyed theirs. Certainly he didn't feel deprived: Everyone ate what he wanted, they all respected each other for this—and they all had a good time.

If people see that you're serious about yourself and your program, but that you can laugh about it and be flexible, they'll do their best to help you. But most of all, the atmosphere will be so positive that you can't help succeeding.

Cocktail parties

A cocktail party is something that takes place before dinner, in the afternoon, at some time other than mealtime.

Go to the cocktail party! Don't deprive yourself of the fun. Just remember! We don't eat between meals.

What a relief to know before you go to a cocktail party that you don't have to make any decisions. You're just not going to eat anything! You can have a club soda or water or tea or coffee, but there isn't anything else you can have. Stay away from the tables with the food on them. Try not to even look at them. Remember, you are a person who doesn't eat between meals, therefore, you don't eat at cocktail parties. Not even a radish. The worst mistake of all would be to have a taste of anything. It just makes the palate want more.

Be kind to yourself. Go to the cocktail parties. You're not giving up a good time—you're just not eating between meals. A cocktail party is a time to get together with friends and have fun. Life is more than one eating experience after another. It's people, and conversation and friendship.

Card parties

On the assumption that this is a party where lunch will be served, the same principle goes for this meal as for eating at a friend's house or at a restaurant. Call your hostess at least a day before you go. "What are you planning to serve? I need to know, as I am on a special diet."

Listen to what she has to say and if you can't eat any of it, ask her if she would mind if you brought your own lunch or if you came after lunch. Frankly, I think it might be more fun for you if you brought your own lunch. Take it to your hostess' kitchen and put it on the same plates she's using. That way, you'll get served with the others but there will be no problems.

Of course, if your hostess could easily adapt her menu to suit you that is a lovely solution. The important thing is to be open about your program, share it, talk about it —make sure the talk stays positive for you.

As for the rest of the time at the card party: the nuts on the table, the perfect mints, the pretzels at your elbow —eat nothing. Take not one taste. You don't eat between meals. You are kind to yourself. One bite of anything will make you crazy. Drink diet soda, chew nonsugared gum, but don't eat anything.

Go and have fun—because you're a person in control of your life, a person who's on top of the world, on your way to the kind of happiness you've always wanted.

The poker game
(or canasta, or whatever your game is)
at your place

Nobody wants to give up the poker game, nor should anyone. But whether it's at a friend's or at your house you should do only what you can handle.

If you're giving the gathering and your friends are used to the big fat sandwiches and beer, and Lord knows what else, you're going to have to decide if you can handle the situation in your own house. Can you indeed deal with everyone gorging themselves on all that stuff, or will you not survive? If you can't survive, then you have a hard task in front of you. You've got to tell them that you can't and ask if they can do without that kind of food for your sake. It's a tough one, but a few of them could probably do with less food themselves. If you can deal with their eating it, then get them what they're used to, but maybe instead of serving it, put the food out on a counter out of your sight, perhaps even in the kitchen, and let them serve themselves.

Remember, the point of the get-together is to play cards not to have food. So concentrate on your game—you'll come out a winner in more ways than one.

The movie theater

Popcorn? What's that? Just something to make your fingers greasy and stick in your teeth. Something other people eat and make too much noise eating.

The movies? What's that? A wonderful form of relaxation. You deserve ninety minutes of calm, uninterrupted, concentrated pleasure. Go to the movies often—and leave your eating at home.

The weekend vacation

First of all, plan to go somewhere where activities are oriented toward anything other than food. Some vacation spots exist only for their cuisine.

No matter what kind of place, get information about the menu before you go. Have it sent to you or discuss it on the phone. Talk to the proprietors about your needs. You will be amazed at how cooperative they can be.

Then, even though you may think the idea a total bore, sit down and plan your menus for the weekend before you leave home. You will have new foods to choose from and think about and work into your program. With your trusty calorie book beside you, you can plan some lovely holiday meals on the basis of what you've learned in advance.

Now go on your weekend, participate in all the activities offered you, except marathon eating. Enjoy yourself. You are a wonderful person who deserves a good time.

The longer vacation

It is possible to take a vacation and continue to lose weight. What you need to pack is "control."

Decide if you want to lose weight on your vacation or just maintain your weight. (Surely the third option, wanting to gain weight, is out of the question, right?) If you want to continue to lose weight, then simply go on doing what you've been doing. Stay on the program.

If you want more leeway, and have decided only to maintain your weight, then add about three hundred to five hundred calories a day to your calorie guide and put the same systems into effect.

(1) Stay in control.

(2) Know what you're going to eat in advance.

(3) Keep your diary going.

(4) Try to weigh yourself every day to make certain the added calories are indeed maintaining your weight rather than increasing it.

(5) Try new foods and new combinations if the calories are within your limits.

(6) Concentrate on activities other than eating.

(7) Enjoy your vacation and yourself.

(8) Come home knowing you're in control of your life, and go back to your calorie allotment for your weight-losing period.

The middle-of-the-night trip to the refrigerator

If you are someone who gets up at two in the morning and sneaks to the kitchen, this is for you.

You're behaving this way primarily because you're dry in the mouth. You need something cold. Perhaps your sinuses are bothering you.

You must keep your refrigerator stocked with diet soda or iced tea or sparkling bottled spring water. Keep those things in the front of the refrigerator shelves, visible, easily available.

Then take one of your "good" crystal glasses. Pour the spring water, for example, over ice and add some fresh lime or lemon. Imagine you're sitting at the most romantic, plush bar in Paris. How elegant, how cool, what a treat.

Now go back to bed, and in the morning when you step on the scale, you will find that life has continued in the positive way you've set out to achieve.

The golf course – eating out at the nineteenth hole

It's hot, you're tired, you're hungry. Are you sure you wouldn't rather invite everyone back to your place for lunch? You prefer the clubhouse, the restaurant, the "nineteenth hole?" Then do it, but make sure you've planned it. What do they have that you can eat? Hard-boiled eggs, salad, shrimp, tuna fish, unsweetened iced tea? Just check, plan your meal, pull up a chair and enjoy your gang, your day, your life. Mark down in your diary and on your score card that the nineteenth hole was a hole-in-one for you today.

The street fair, the county fair

If your fairs are the same as the ones I know, they should be called food fairs.

My suggestion is, Don't go this year! There is too little to alleviate the pressure. Food is the primary purpose of the fair. Be kind to yourself. Go somewhere else this year where *you* can have fun!

The ball game or sporting event

How can you possibly go without eating the hot dogs?

There's only one way: by telling yourself that next year you will, but today you have a job to do.

You don't eat between meals. You didn't come here to eat. You came to watch your favorite sport, so shout and scream and have a good time.

You don't need the food to have a good time. All you need is for your team to go out there and do its best.

Making it through the holidays: Christmas, Easter, Passover, Thanksgiving, etc.

We do get tested in many ways in our lives, but holidays are really the supreme test. The first thing you have to say to yourself is that it's only for *this* Christmas, *this* Passover, *this* Thanksgiving—not forever. So if we can just get through this one holiday, it will mean that the next time it rolls around we will have accomplished our purpose and can take a few little liberties with our lives.

YOU ARE MORE SPECIAL THAN THE SPECIAL HOLIDAY. Remember that, and you'll stay on the program. Now let's take a practical approach to the holiday.

Thanksgiving

This is the hardest one for most people. Other holidays have special events associated with them—ritual or church or trees or presents—but Thanksgiving means just one thing: EATING. Rather, it's two things: PREPARING AND EATING.

If you're the one who ordinarily prepares the Thanksgiving meal, think about whether it is possible to farm it out this year or to make arrangements to share the cooking with someone else. Perhaps you can make the turkey and your guests can do the other things. If you can work this out, you will be doing yourself a favor, because getting through the preparation of all those goodies—and not eating—requires extraordinary strength.

Remember, we're trying to be kind to ourselves, and being involved in that kitchen for a day or two is unkind —cruel, in fact. If you can't get out of it, then take precautions: make sure there is someone in the kitchen helping

—who knows you're on a special program. This will prevent you from tasting everything. They can do the tasting for you. Remember: if they asked you for help, you would do anything you could. Have confidence that they will respond the same way.

If all else fails, and you can't get anyone to be with you during the preparation, then here's a bizarre and ridiculous suggestion that works. Get yourself one of those surgical masks they use in hospitals. Put it on, and you will find that it is almost impossible to get any food into your mouth without pulling it off—which you'll feel inhibited about. If anyone laughs at you while you're wearing it, don't be on the defensive. Laugh too. After all, even though it's serious stuff, it's funny. But at the same time . . . you're staying in control.

As to the eating part of Thanksgiving, the best thing you could do for yourself would be put your head into a hole in the floor or into the oven or lock yourself in the linen closet until the whole thing is over. But we're grownups, and we can and will face this thing. The second-best thing to do is just what you always do. Write down in your diary at least the day before exactly what you can eat and still stay within your calorie count. When dinnertime comes around, eat only that.

Sounds too simple, doesn't it? Well, it is simple. What we're doing is leaving out the compulsive, impulsive things we do about eating. We are protecting ourselves with the calm, reasoned decisions we made the day before when we weren't being bombarded with the smells and sights of food all around us.

The number-57th-best thing to do about Thanksgiving —and this suggestion is only if you know in your heart

of hearts that you will succumb when you get to the table
—is to write it down the day before so that you will keep
in control. If your calorie count is 400 for the meal, figure
about 300 calories and write the foods down.

Then list, in writing, each and every dish that will be
available on that groaning board. Write this list with the
words *one teaspoon* before each entry. In other words,
write: *one teaspoon* of sweet potatoes, *one teaspoon* of
stuffing, *one teaspoon* of mashed potatoes, *one teaspoon* of
pumpkin pie. At the table, take 300 calories of what you
know you can eat, and then take a teaspoon of everything
else that is offered. Put it on your plate ahead of time, just
like you do all your meals. This is what you are going to
eat, no more, no less. You will have tasted everything.
You will have plenty to eat. You will not have more than
you just put on your plate. You are a person on your way
to thinhood, in control even during Thanksgiving and
having a terrific time. You can tell yourself: I am a terrific
person who has used the 57th-best thing to help myself
over a severe problem. I have done it beautifully, by staying in control.

Passover

The only thing that would differ at all for this holiday
concerns the food that must be eaten during the ceremony. Eat it. It's just not enough to worry about. If your
conscience dictates that you go through the ceremony,
eating the ceremonial food, then go through it. But keep
the food in perspective. Write even this down the day
before in your diary, and when it comes to the meal do
the same thing as for Thanksgiving: only resort to the
"57th solution" if you can't deal with just eating your
planned 400 calories.

Christmas

Dealing with Christmas has the added complication of gifts. How often do you give gifts that are food? How often do you take presents to people's homes that are food? How often do you present food to people you care about?

Think about this—and think about not doing it any more. There are wonderful presents to be given that have nothing to do with food, that don't require your going into food departments for gifts, or cheese stores for the perfect cheese. You don't have to put yourself through the excruciating torment of having to deal with such sights and smells, or with carrying such a time-bomb present around with you. Give plants, books, lovely glasses.

There's an interesting parallel here. An Alcoholics Anonymous member recently observed that, before they became members of A.A., every time A.A. people went anywhere they gave a bottle of liquor. All their presents were alcoholic. It's the same for many of us, but it's a habit and a hazard that is easily discarded. Not bringing food is being kind to yourself—and to the people you're gifting.

General Advice About Holidays, Ceremonies and Special Occasions

First of all, *go to them*. Enjoy them and keep the food in the proper perspective. These are not occasions merely for the consumption of food, although perhaps that's where your head has always been. They are times for celebration, times to be with people you genuinely care about and who care about you. Be happy that your world is filled with these good times and these good people. Go and put the food on your plate, not in your heart.

If you choose the "57th solution" discussed under Thanksgiving, understand that you are still in charge of your life. You are not a victim of special occasions—you enjoy them.

Chapter IX

The Food Program!
The Diet!

We've spent our time together learning how to live with food—now we're going to talk about what to eat and how much. The diet that seems to work best on this program is based on 700 calories for the day. Seven hundred is not sacrosanct; you may choose 800 or 900 or 1000, depending on what makes you feel most comfortable and the rate at which you lose weight. Also, as we have discussed, before you launch on this diet—or any other diet—consult with your doctor.

	700-calorie diet	800-calorie diet	900-calorie diet	1000-calorie diet
Breakfast	150	200	200	250
Lunch	150	200	250	250
Dinner	400	400	450	500
	700	800	900	1000

On the 700-calorie diet, women should lose an average of 2 to 2 1/2 pounds a week. For men, it will average more —about 3 to 3 1/2 pounds a week. The more calories you decided to eat, the slower your rate of loss will be. Find what makes you comfortable and stick with it. Consistency is everything.

Also, try to balance carbohydrates and protein. Take a good multiple vitamin with minerals every day.

The food breakdown for each meal is as follows:

	700 calories	800 calories	900 calories	1000 calories
BREAKFAST				
1/3 calories—dairy (skimmed milk, cottage cheese, egg whites)	(approx.) 50	70	70	90
1/3 calories—cereals, breads	50	65	65	80
1/3 calories—fruit (fresh, canned, juice)	50	65	65	80
	150	200	200	250
LUNCH				
2/3 calories—skimmed milk, egg whites, cottage cheese, tuna fish, shrimp, chicken	100	130	165	165
1/3 calories—salad greens, vegetables, fruits, breads	50	70	85	85
	150	200	250	250
DINNER				
2/3–3/4 calories—chicken, fish, beef, cottage cheese, skimmed milk	265–300	265–300	300–325	330–375
1/3–1/4 calories—vegetables, salads, fruits	135–100	135–100	150–125	170–125
	400	400	450	500
TOTALS	700	800	900	1000

After you have studied this diet, go back to the beginning of the book, especially to the *support system*. This is the time to figure out what your diet is going to be. Take out your diary and write down your first meal. Use your calorie book to help you figure out what you can have. Measure yourself, write the information down and begin.

Take a deep breath. Just feel how wonderful it is to be alive and ready to move onto another place in life. It is a place where we can feel respect for ourselves, where we can have hope again. And this time we will do it right.

The nutritious and satisfying breakfast

150 Calories

Breakfast at home:

1/4 cup of cottage cheese	50–60 calories
1/4 cup of bran cereal (1 ounce)	60–70 calories
1/3 cup of sliced peaches or 1-1/2 peach halves or 1/3 cup of fruit cocktail	30 calories
Tea or coffee	
	approx. 150 calories

Allow yourself a good twenty minutes to eat this breakfast. It is bulky and chewy and satisfying. I add sweetener and vanilla and cinnamon. Some find it sweet enough as is.

An alternative could be fried egg whites. Separate the eggs and dispose of the yolks, unless you know someone who just loves cholesterol. Use a Teflon pan or spray a pan with a no-calorie, no-stick spray. Beat the whites a bit and toss them in a pan. In minutes, you will have lovely fried eggs—to which you could add onions or cottage cheese or peaches.

112

3 egg whites	45 calories
2 slices of onion	5
1 ounce of bran cereal	60
1/4 cup skimmed milk	40
	150

4 egg whites	60 calories
1/4 cup of cottage cheese	50
1/2 cup of peaches	40
	150

With the advent of low-calorie preserves, you could make yourself a delicious crepe or blintzes, using the egg whites, stuffing the "pancake" with cottage cheese and dotting it with strawberry or peach preserves at 2 calories a teaspoon. Delicious. Put that in the back of your mind for a possible quick dessert or even a nice luncheon dish when friends are visiting.

Think of breakfast as just as important as any other meal of the day. Use this time to get the day's events straight. Plan the day, structure your time.

The kind and delicious lunch

150 calories

Lunch at home:

A wonderful salad

2 ounces of tuna (water-packed)	60 calories
3 hard-boiled egg whites	45
2 cups of mixed salad greens	20
A couple of slices of onion or scallion	5
Diet dressing	20
	150 calories

113

Quick tuna salad

2 ounces of tuna	60 calories
1/4 cup of cottage cheese	50
2 slices of tomato	20
2 slices of onion	5
	135 calories

Combination salad and vegetable lunch

2 ounces of tuna	60 calories
1 slice of tomato	10
2 cups of salad	20
Onion	5
Diet dressing	20
1 cup of cooked cauliflower	30
(or broccoli or summer squash or	
green beans)	
	145 calories

Egg-white omelet

4 egg whites	60 calories
1/2 cup of mushrooms	25
1/4 cup of cottage cheese	50
2 slices of tomato	20
	155 calories

Fry the egg whites in a Teflon pan. Heat the mushrooms and stir in the cottage cheese. Add paprika and pour the mixture into the omelet. Slide onto your plate and garnish with the tomato.

Other omelettes could contain onions and mushrooms, onions and green peppers and mushrooms, zucchini and tomatoes.

Lunch at the office:

Keep 3½-ounce cans of water-packed tuna at your desk. Then order from the coffee shop some garden salad without dressing.

You can bring in cottage cheese and eat that with the

garden salad or even mix the cottage cheese with some all-bran cereal for a delicious crunchy lunch.

Keep it simple, stick to a few basics like tuna fish, cottage cheese, egg whites. Embellish these to please your palate. Good luck! Enjoy!

The luxurious and enviable dinner

400 Calories

Your basics for dinner include chicken, fish and vegetables. If you're a beef fancier, use chopped beef or lean roasts, but be careful of the calories. The better the beef, the higher the fat content and the more the calories. Sirloin steak, for example, can range from 80 to 125 calories an ounce. However, a thin-sliced London Broil can be about the same as chicken, 50 or 50 calories an ounce. Eat what you like, just weigh your food and figure the calories.

Dinner at home:

Breast of chicken (5 1/2 ounces)	275
1 cup of cauliflower	30
1/2 cup of green beans	15
1 cup of tossed salad	10
Diet dressing	30
A peach	35
	395

Breast of chicken	275
1 stalk of broccoli	45
1 cup of squash	30
1 cup of tossed salad	10
Diet dressing	30
	390

We discussed earlier how to cook the chicken: remove the skin, broil on both sides for 5 minutes, then roast, uncovered, for 40 minutes at 350 degrees. Don't cook the vegetables too long. Let them keep their original color and crispness.

Dinner out:

Fish (dry, no butter or oil)	200
Baked potato	100
1 cup of tossed salad	10
Diet dressing	10
1/4 cup of spinach	10
10 fresh strawberries	35
	365

Try putting the spinach into the baked potato. It's better than butter!

As you can see, 400 calories go a long way for dinner. You can have a wonderful meal, with courses like everyone else. There will be plenty of food to eat, and you will feel neither like a glutton nor deprived.

Enjoy your new food program. It's easy, it's good and it's ready to take you where you want to go: on the road to being a thin person in charge of life.

Chapter X

You Can Have
Wines and Liquors!

If wine is something you want in your life while on your program, consider it as another food. It has calories, just as a soft drink does.

As long as the wine or liquor doesn't exceed 10 percent of your calories for the day, you've got it in perspective, both calorically, psychologically and nutritionally. Therefore on 700 calories for the day you can have 70 calories of wine or liquor. Be careful, though, about which wine you're consuming. Dessert wines are very high in calories and would not be affordable on your program. Most dry wines average about 25 calories an ounce, and most wine glasses contain about 4 ounces. Fill the glass about three-quarters of the way and you'll be fine. Make sure you don't deprive yourself of your protein calories—for wine or anything else. Wine does contain some vitamins and certain good psychological attributes.

As for cooking with wine, as long as you're using the regular 25-calories-per-ounce wines, you can be rather confident that most of the calories will burn up in the cooking. If, however, you are using the highly caloric dessert wines, the sugar content will definitely remain and, therefore, the calories. Moderation is the order of the day. Be careful, but if you plan it, and it works in your program, enjoy it.

As for liquor, the caloric value of liquors depends on their proof. The higher the proof, the higher the calories. For 1½ ounces of liquor (a jigger's worth):

Proof	Calories
80	100
90	110
100	125

That's a lot of calories for a little bit of stuff. But it can be done, as long as it is planned for and counted and is a PART OF YOUR MEAL. The same goes for wine. Remember, calories are food whether you're eating them or drinking them and WE ARE PEOPLE WHO DO NOT EAT BE-TWEEN MEALS. Therefore, wine or liquor cannot be taken at a cocktail party or at any time except at meals.

For those of you who enjoy or endure business lunches, the cocktail or glass of wine may seem to be imperative. If it is, plan for it and have it. However, these days, many people don't drink at lunch or, if they do, drink club soda or spring water, with a twist of lemon or lime. If you find you want a drink, you can deal with one. Again, figure your calories. Perhaps you'll have to permanently adjust the calorie distribution for the day, taking more for lunch, slightly fewer for dinner.

Remember to watch out for the calories in mixers like ginger ale, tonic or Coke. You're in control here, not the food or drink.

Chapter XI

Once You Have Become
a Thin Person or
Almost a Thin Person

The most dangerous time for all of us is when we have *almost* reached our goal. That is because we are special. We are different. We may indeed become thin persons, but we never are thin inside. We can never let go, believe we're just like anyone else and therefore eat like anyone else. We can't. Don't make this mistake. We must stay in control of our food and in control of its place in our life ... *all our life.*

This shouldn't depress you. Knowing that there is a solution to your problem should give you great joy. Think how lucky you are that you are dealing with something that can be fixed. It's not like some dread disease that has no cure or leaves an unfixable impediment. Your special problem just requires your diligence.

When you're on your way to being thin, you must find a food maintenance level for yourself. If you stay on the 700-, 800-, 900-, or 1000-a-day calories for two months, then go on maintenance at 1200 to 1500 calories for two months—it gives your body a chance to adjust each time to a new level. During the maintenance period, don't go on the scale every day. Try once a week, until you see that your weight is being stabilized. Then go back to your dieting for another two months and continue the pattern till you reach your goal. By this time, you will have found out how many calories you need to consume to maintain your weight. Experiment, but I think you'll find that you need a lot fewer calories to maintain your weight than you expected. You will also find out that after having eaten 700 to 1000 calories a day for two months, 1200 to 1500 will seem an enormous amount of food.

Remember, you are not like anyone else. Your body may become thin, but it will always have a disposition to fill up again. You must, you can, you will—stay in control. Don't waste the months, the days, the hours, the minutes that you have spent being kind to yourself by thinking that once you see this thin person in the mirror, this person will automatically stay thin for life. You have, while becoming thin, learned wonderful things about yourself:

You are a special person!
You are someone who is kind to yourself!
You protect yourself!
You are not a victim!
You are in control of your life!
You are terrific!

Chapter XII

The Sample Diary

Day	Weight in A.M.	Mood in Morning
Friday, 6/1	160	Good

Before-Breakfast Reminders	*Yes*	*No*
1. Have you planned your meals?	X	
2. Have you planned your day's activities?		
If not, do it now.	X	
3. Have you got your shopping list?	X	
4. Have you reread your commandments?	X	
5. Have you told yourself you're terrific?	X	
6. Have you weighed yourself?	X	

Breakfast

Where ____Home____ With whom ___By myself___	*Planned Calories*	*Unplanned Calories*
1 ounce of bran cereal	60	
1/4 cup of cottage cheese	50	
1/2 cup of peaches (2 halves)	40	
TOTAL	150	0

Activities Between Breakfast and Lunch   *Mood*

Grocery shopping	or	Arrived at office	Felt good—really
Cleaned the house		Advertising meeting	on top of it—a
Took dry cleaning		Coffee break	good day begin-
Did laundry		Worked at desk	ning.

Lunch

Where _At desk or Home_ With whom ____By myself____	*Planned Calories*	*Unplanned Calories*
2 cups of salad	20	
2 ounces of tuna (water-packed)	60	
3 hard-boiled egg whites	45	
2 slices of tomato	15	
Onion	5	
Low-calorie Italian dressing	10	
TOTAL	155	0

Activities Between Lunch and Dinner   *Mood*

Stopped at record
  store
	or	Met agent to go over
		  book
			Feeling good and
			productive.

Saw paper sales-
  man
		Went to Y for meet-
		  ing on Boy Scouts	

Worked at desk		Picked up jeans (new size)	

122

Dinner

| Where _____Hobeau's_____ | *Planned* | *Unplanned* |
| With whom _____Richard_____ | *Calories* | *Calories* |

Filet of sole (7 ounces)	210	
Baked potato	100	
Salad	30	
My dressing	35	
Broccoli	15	
TOTAL	390	0

Activities Between Dinner and Sleep	*Mood*
Dinner lasted till 10:30 P.M.	Lovely dinner—
Home, watched TV till 11:30.	and I felt calm! A
Read till 12:30	truly productive
	day 'cause I was
	in control!

Day's total planned	*Day's total unplanned*
calories	*calories*
695	0

How Much Exercise Have You Had Today?   *Walked about two miles.*

Before bed	*Yes*	*No*
1. Are tomorrow's meals planned?	X	
2. Have you planned your activities for tomorrow?	X	

Feelings About Yourself and the Day. Express Yourself!

I can't get over the calm that I feel. It's so good to know that I'm prepared for today, tomorrow and the next day. I know I can handle it all. I feel so much better about myself and about the people around me. I love being able to cross my legs under the dining room table while eating! I can't wait until tomorrow.

The Diary

Day   *Weight in* A.M.   *Mood in Morning*

Before-Breakfast Reminders   *Yes*   *No*

1. Have you planned your meals?
2. Have you planned your day's activities?
    If not, do it now.
3. Have you got your shopping list?
4. Have you reread your commandments?
5. Have you told yourself you're terrific?
6. Have you weighed yourself?

reakfast

Where _____   *Planned*   *Unplanned*
With whom _____   *Calories*   *Calories*

Activities Between Breakfast and Lunch   *Mood*

Lunch

Where _____   *Planned*   *Unplanned*
With whom _____   *Calories*   *Calories*

Activities Between Lunch and Dinner   *Mood*

Dinner

Where _____   *Planned*   *Unplanned*
With whom _____   *Calories*   *Calories*

Activities Between Dinner and Sleep   *Mood*

Day's total planned   *Day's total unplanned*
calories   *calories*

How Much Exercise Have You Had Today?   _____ _____

Before bed   *Yes*   *No*

1. Are tomorrow's meals planned?
2. Have you planned your activities
    for tomorrow?

Feelings About Yourself and the Day. Express Yourself!

127

The Diary

Day   *Weight in* A.M.   *Mood in Morning*

Before-Breakfast Reminders   *Yes*   *No*

1. Have you planned your meals?
2. Have you planned your day's activities?
   If not, do it now.
3. Have you got your shopping list?
4. Have you reread your commandments?
5. Have you told yourself you're terrific?
6. Have you weighed yourself?

Breakfast

Where _____   *Planned*   *Unplanned*
With whom _____   *Calories*   *Calories*

Activities Between Breakfast and Lunch   *Mood*

Lunch

Where _____   *Planned*   *Unplanned*
With whom _____   *Calories*   *Calories*

Activities Between Lunch and Dinner   *Mood*

Dinner

Where _____   *Planned*   *Unplanned*
With whom _____   *Calories*   *Calories*

130

Activities Between Dinner and Sleep   *Mood*

Day's total planned   *Day's total unplanned*
calories   *calories*

How Much Exercise Have You Had Today?   _____ _____

Before bed   *Yes*   *No*

1. Are tomorrow's meals planned?
2. Have you planned your activities
   for tomorrow?

Feelings About Yourself and the Day. Express Yourself!

The Diary

Day   *Weight in* A.M.   *Mood in Morning*

Before-Breakfast Reminders   *Yes*   *No*

1. Have you planned your meals?
2. Have you planned your day's activities?
   If not, do it now.
3. Have you got your shopping list?
4. Have you reread your commandments?
5. Have you told yourself you're terrific?
6. Have you weighed yourself?

Breakfast

Where _____   *Planned*   *Unplanned*
With whom _____   *Calories*   *Calories*

Activities Between Breakfast and Lunch   *Mood*

Lunch

Where _____   *Planned*   *Unplanned*
With whom _____   *Calories*   *Calories*

Activities Between Lunch and Dinner   *Mood*

Dinner

Where _____   *Planned*   *Unplanned*
With whom _____   *Calories*   *Calories*

Activities Between Dinner and Sleep　　　　　　*Mood*

　　　　Day's total planned　　　*Day's total unplanned*
　　　　　　calories　　　　　　　　*calories*

How Much Exercise Have You Had Today?　　　_____

Before bed　　　　　　　　　　　　*Yes*　　　　*No*

1. Are tomorrow's meals planned?
2. Have you planned your activities
　　for tomorrow?

Feelings About Yourself and the Day. Express Yourself!

About the Author

During the past twenty years RAYSA ROSE BONOW has been a pioneer in television broadcasting, one of the first women managers in her field. She is a native of Westmont, in Pennsylvania, and now lives in a garden apartment in Manhattan. Ms. Bonow is currently at work on two new books on pet care.